FITNESS:
A LIFETIME COMMITMENT

David K. Miller
T. Earl Allen

University of North Carolina
Wilmington, North Carolina

Burgess Publishing Company
Minneapolis, Minnesota

Cover design and photograph by Lynn Guilfoyle Dwyer.

Copyright © 1979 by Burgess Publishing Company
Printed in the United States of America
Library of Congress Catalog Card Number 78-67970
ISBN 0-8087-3935-2

0 9 8 7 6 5 4 3

To our wives, Roselyn and Johanna

PREFACE

This book is designed primarily for college men and women enrolled in courses in physical fitness, body conditioning, or foundations of physical activity. The objectives are to provide a meaningful understanding of the purpose of physical exercise, to enable the student to evaluate his or her own level of physical fitness, and to design a personalized exercise program that can be beneficial throughout life.

Throughout this book, the word *exercise* and the term *exercise program* will be used. Unless otherwise stated, both are interpreted to mean an organized, regular program of physical activity designed to develop or maintain the components of physical fitness.

Some authors define *physical fitness* as the capacity for sustained physical activity without excessive fatigue or as the capacity to perform everyday activities with reserve energy for emergency situations. Many individuals may incorrectly classify themselves as physically fit by these definitions, and it is especially incorrect to accept these definitions when the relations between inactivity and health are considered. For the purposes of this book, no definition of physical fitness will be given. However, the concept will be taken to include circulorespiratory endurance, muscular strength and endurance, flexibility, and weight management.

Key terms, the pages on which they are found, and behavioral objectives are listed at the beginning of each chapter. Fulfillment of these objectives will accomplish the purposes of the book. The key terms appear in boldface roman type, and other words that the authors wish to emphasize are italicized.

Each chapter is designed to stand alone, and the sequence of chapters may be rearranged to meet the needs of a particular group of students. To develop a meaningful understanding of heart disease, exercise prescription, and training responses to exercise, the student should possess a basic knowledge of the anatomy and physiology of the circulatory, respiratory, and muscular systems. Chapters 8, 9, and 10 include this information for the student whose background is inadequate. However, important concepts other than those of basic anatomy and physiology are also included in those chapters.

The appendix includes a test for self-evaluation of circulorespiratory endurance, a table for physical fitness classification, and percentile score for Cooper's Twelve-Minute Run. A glossary is provided for clarificat~ terms not fully defined in the text.

The authors wish to express their appreciation to the m~ and colleagues who directly and indirectly have contribute~

of this book and to the publishers who have graciously allowed the reproduction of tables. Most grateful acknowledgment is also extended to Sharon Brewington for her assistance in the preparation of the manuscript, to Talmsi Schultz and Jan Allen for the illustrations, and to Dillon Bryant and Chuck Chance for the photography. David Cameron, T. L. Doolittle, A. W. Faris, Ed Hooks, Marylou Morgan, and Doug Smith are thanked for their early reviews of the manuscript. A special debt is owed to Bob Clayton for assistance and encouragement throughout the project.

TABLE OF CONTENTS

10 THE MUSCULAR SYSTEM, POSTURE, AND MOVEMENT MECHANICS 131

11 SUMMARY 145

GLOSSARY 151

INDEX 155

LABORATORY SESSIONS 159

KEY TERMS
Body image (p. 2)
Hypokinetic disease (p. 3)
Neuromuscular efficiency (p. 3)
Self-concept (p. 2)
Self-estimate (p. 2)
Self-image (p. 2)

BEHAVIORAL OBJECTIVES
Upon completion of this chapter, the student should be able to:
1. Define the key terms listed above.
2. Describe five major changes and problems that the human population has experienced in modern times.
3. List and discuss at least six benefits to be gained from a regular exercise program.

CHAPTER ONE
INTRODUCTION

People are designed for physical activity. Primitive humans had to be able to run, climb, jump, and throw to provide for their needs and to escape constant threats to their lives. They had to be physically fit: only the fittest survived. This capacity for physical activity remains present in modern people. Even the developing embryo moves within the uterus long before the mother becomes aware of it. After the infant is born, the parents can hardly wait for the child to crawl and walk, but encouragement to move is not really needed: the desire to walk, skip, run, and play is present from the start. Often during adolescence and adulthood, however, habits of inactivity are developed and permitted to become a part of daily living.

The development of these habits of inactivity is primarily due to the presence of labor-saving devices. One hundred years ago, only 6% of the energy used to produce goods was mechanical; the remaining 94% was generated by human or animal muscle power. Today, however, as much as 96% of all energy used is mechanical. Power steering and power brakes, riding lawn mowers, remote-control television, and similar devices have made the American people weaker and lazier. Associated with this life-style have been increases in the number of people experiencing degenerative and cardiovascular diseases, excessive weight gain, lower back pain, and mental illness. Also, the **self-concept, self-image, body image,** and **self-estimate** of many individuals have suffered due to lack of movement and physical deterioration.

In addition, the population of today has experienced more changes and crises than has any other generation. The knowledge explosion and the use of computers, the population explosion, increased leisure time, the energy crisis, pollution, and the frenzied pace of living are but a few of the major changes and problems facing the world today. These changes and crises have altered the human environment much too fast. Mental strain and stress have resulted, creating a way of life that is biologically and psychologically unsuitable. To compensate for the daily pressures that they must face, people depend on coffee to awaken them in the morning, alcohol and tranquilizers to calm their disturbed nerves, and sleeping pills to help them rest at night. However, these drinks and pills have not succeeded in providing the desired results: mental illness is more prevalent now than ever before.

Even though these habits of inactivity have developed and our environment has changed, the very important and basic human need for movement has remained. Movement is refreshing: the simple act of opening and closing the hand or tapping the foot can be a relief to someone who must remain sitting or standing for a long period of time. The morning and afternoon breaks from one's work are often refreshing due to the moving or walking associated with them. Movement is necessary even during sleep to promote circulation.

Movement is also related to one's self-concept. Self-image, body image, and self-estimate constitute self-concept; an individual who ranks low on any one of them will probably have a poor self-concept. A successful exercise program can improve one's self-image and self-estimate. Also, movement and action are essential for the development of one's body image.

An individual who has a healthy body image, self-image, and self-estimate is more likely to attempt new physical activities, and participation in these can provide opportunities for social recognition and development of friendships. Various group activities can also develop one's ability to work harmoniously with other individuals and to adjust to their wishes and feelings. Often a togetherness of the group emerges and carries over into situations other than those found in sports. Many individuals fail to enjoy the social interaction that can be experienced in a program of physical activity due to their unwarranted concern about physical appearance and performance and their low estimate of potential success. A specified level of physical fitness, which in turn may improve one's self-concept, should be developed prior to participation in leisure activities if maximum social benefits are to be gained from this participation.

Perhaps an even more important aspect of movement is the possible prevention of degenerative and cardiovascular diseases. The law of use and disuse dictates that one must use one's body if it is to be developed and maintained at a high level of efficiency, and that, if one fails to do so, the body will deteriorate (**hypokinetic disease**). There is more and more evidence to indicate that a regular exercise program keeps the cardiovascular system, as well as other systems of the body, in good condition. Exercise develops the heart and lungs, so that they are able to supply oxygen to the muscles without strain. Regular exercise has been reported to improve coronary circulation and to reduce the risk of obstructive arterial disease. An exercise program helps one maintain desirable weight, and it also helps prevent the weight gain, lower back pain, loss of flexibility, and other degenerative diseases often associated with aging. Improvement in muscular strength and endurance, blood supply, innervation, and flexibility enhance **neuromuscular efficiency,** which increases the participant's chances for success in leisure activities.

In addition, emotional needs are related to the need for movement. The human body has identical reactions to mental and physical stress. This means that a physically fit individual is better prepared to adapt to and cope with mental stress. Physical activity provides an outlet that enables an individual to "let go," to release instinctive aggressive drives, and to relieve pent-up emotions of anger and hostility. The mental peace and physical relaxation that usually follow an exercise session enhance the participant's emotional health. Many Americans would be well advised to seek peace and relaxation this way rather than through alcohol or drugs.

From all the reasons given here, it should be apparent that a regular physical exercise program is not a luxury but a necessity. There are many types and variations of exercise programs, and each individual should select one according to personal interests and needs. However, everyone should know the why, as well as the how, of physical exercise. If individuals truly understand its purpose, more will follow a regular exercise regimen.

KEY TERMS
Angina pectoris (p. 7)
Atherosclerosis (p. 6)
Coronary heart disease (CHD) (p. 6)
Fibrous plaque (p. 8)
High-density lipoprotein (HDL) (p. 11)
Hypercholesterolemia (p. 10)
Hyperlipemia (p. 10)
Hypertension (p. 10)
Ischemia (p. 6)
Low-density lipoprotein (LDL) (p. 11)
Myocardial infarction (p. 7)
Regurgitation murmur (p. 13)
Serum cholesterol (p. 10)
Serum triglycerides (p. 10)
Stenosis (p. 13)

BEHAVIORAL OBJECTIVES
Upon completion of this chapter, the student should be able to:
1. Define the key terms listed above.
2. Identify two theories that seek to explain the origin and development of atherosclerosis.
3. List the steps in the progressive development of coronary heart disease in terms of the multifactorial theory.
4. Identify the primary and secondary risk factors that the multifactorial theory associates with the development of coronary heart disease.
5. Identify safe ranges for blood pressure and safe levels for serum cholesterol and serum triglycerides.
6. Discuss the role of exercise in the prevention of and the rehabilitation after coronary heart disease.

CHAPTER TWO
HEART DISEASE

Basic knowledge of causes, preventive measures, and modern treatments should result in reduced anxiety about the prospects of heart disease. In addition, this knowledge should enable the reader to respond intelligently to personal problems that might occur at some future date. Due to the limited scope of this manual, only a few of the more common types of heart disorders are described, as follows:

1. Coronary heart disease (resulting in angina pectoris or myocardial infarction)
2. Valvular lesions
3. Rhythm disorders
4. Congenital defects

CORONARY HEART DISEASE

By far the most important disease of the heart and vascular system, at least in terms of premature death or reduced quality of life, is **coronary heart disease** (**CHD**). Of the deaths attributable to diseases of the heart, CHD annually claims the lives of over 700,000 Americans. Forty percent of all deaths in men between the ages of 40 and 59 are the result of CHD. The American Heart Association estimated that 52% of all deaths in the United States in 1977 were due to some form of cardiovascular disease. (See Figure 2-1.)

The economic impact of CHD in this country is tremendous. In 1970, medical expenses, losses due to time spent away from work, and related costs amounted to $25 billion. By 1973, that figure had risen to $40 billion. It has been estimated that, with inflation and the increasing incidence of CHD, the cost in 1977 came close to $50 billion.

Atherosclerosis

Atherosclerosis is a major contributor to the development of CHD. It is a progressive condition, developing over a long period of time, not something that appears suddenly one morning in middle age. The etiology of atherosclerosis is very controversial. Whatever the cause, *lesions* develop in the walls of the coronary arteries. Over the years, this pathologic process continues until the blood flow is seriously reduced (a condition known as **ischemia**) or even until the vessel becomes completely occluded. The slowly developing atherosclerotic process finally becomes dramatically manifest in the occurrence of angina pectoris or myocardial infarction (heart attack).

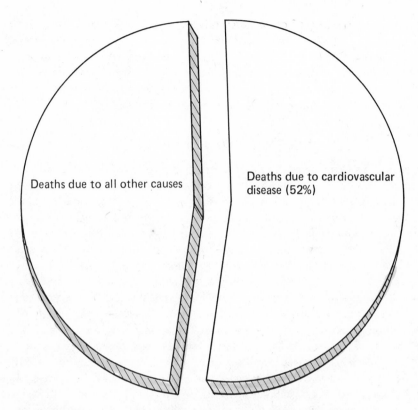

Deaths due to all other causes

Deaths due to cardiovascular disease (52%)

Figure 2-1. Deaths from cardiovascular disease in the United States in 1977.

Angina Pectoris

The term **angina pectoris** means chest pain. This disorder is caused by an inability of the coronary arteries to supply the myocardium (heart muscle) with oxygen. The pain is usually not present when one is at rest but is precipitated by physical exertion. It is described as excruciating, often radiating from the sternum to the shoulders, jaw, and arms. It usually subsides with the cessation of the activity. Treatment, depending on the severity of the condition, includes drug therapy, exercise, or surgical procedures.

Myocardial Infarction

A **myocardial infarction** is a heart attack. The term *infarct* refers to an area of dead tissue resulting from inadequate circulation in the myocardium. If a coronary artery becomes occluded by a clot (thrombus) or by some other material, the tissue beyond that point is deprived of blood. The tissue dies (necrosis), and the area is permanently damaged. If the damaged area is large enough, the victim dies. A milder condition can be treated successfully, and many patients can be rehabilitated. As is the case with angina pectoris, drug therapy and exercise are important in the recovery of postinfarcted patients.

DEVELOPMENT OF ATHEROSCLEROSIS

Autopsy examination of the coronary arteries of soldiers (whose average age was 22 years) killed in the Korean and Vietnamese conflicts showed evidence of significant atherosclerotic coronary artery disease (60% and 45%, respectively). In the case of the Vietnam data, approximately 5% of those studied had at least one of the three major coronary arteries almost completely occluded or all three vessels involved to a significant degree. These data clearly demonstrate that atherosclerosis is not just a disease of the aged but is manifest early in life.

One of the major efforts in the United States to trace the development of atherosclerosis was begun in 1947 under the direction of the International Atherosclerosis Project. Researchers in this project collected approximately 30,000 aortas and coronary arteries from around the world and made cross-sectional analyses of subjects from birth to age 70. From the data thus collected, the pathologic process of atherosclerosis was established as follows (11):

1. Below age 10:   Fatty streaks first appear in the aorta as the result of *lipid* deposition in the arterial intima (lining).

    This is considered benign, since it appears to occur in populations of children all around the world, regardless of diet, exercise level, or genetic background.

2. Age 10 to 20:   Fatty deposits begin to appear with increasing frequency in the coronary arteries themselves. This occurs particularly in western populations.

3. Age 20 to 40:   The lipid materials continue to build up in the arterial wall until age 35 or 40, when they begin to change into **fibrous plaque** and become covered by fibrous scars.

    Most authorities feel that this development of fibrous plaque marks the point of no return: once plaque formation occurs, the process appears to be irreversible. The process can be somewhat arrested, but the scars will not disappear, as do the fatty streaks.

4. Age 40 and beyond: Finally, the areas of fibrous plaque lead to more complicated lesions involving further lipid deposition, thrombus formation, and eventual death of the tissue beyond the clot.

Until recently, versions of two basic theories have guided investigation of atherosclerosis. The dominant one, the insudation theory, holds that infiltration of lipids from the blood into the artery walls gives rise to cholesterol deposits that act as irritants within the walls and cause further infiltration and proliferation of cells. The other theory, the encrustation theory, holds that plaque begins with a small mural thrombus that is converted into a mass of tissue in the arterial intima as the cells of the arterial wall migrate to it and secrete characteristic extracellular substances (1). Since the mid-1960s, the multifactorial version of the insudation theory, which was developed mostly from epidemiological data, has been the one most widely accepted by the medical profession. Recently, however, a new hypothesis, the monoclonal cell proliferation theory, has been gaining considerable acceptance (1).

Multifactorial Theory

The most widely accepted theory concerning the development of atherosclerosis does not regard any one factor as playing a more dominant role than any other. Rather, research in epidemiology points towards a "multifactorial cause," involving certain primary factors or combinations of factors, as being responsible for increasing one's risk of developing the disease. The following are considered *primary risk factors:*

1. Hypertension (high blood pressure)
2. Hyperlipemia (abnormally high levels of serum triglycerides and/or serum cholesterol in circulating blood)
3. Cigarette smoking

Following closely behind and not necessarily listed in order of importance are these *secondary risk factors:*

4. Obesity
5. Sedentary living habits
6. Psychological or emotional stress
7. *Glucose* intolerance (diabetes mellitus)
8. Positive family history of heart disease
9. Sex

Hypertension

Hypertension (high blood pressure), salt intake, and obesity are all interrelated. Except in extreme cases, blood pressure can be reduced by the control of salt intake, diet, weight, and exercise. In extreme cases, drug therapy becomes necessary and is very effective. It is alarming that medical researchers are seeing higher blood pressures in American children today than in the past. Although it is well known that blood pressure tends to increase with age, there is no reason to accept values higher than those listed.

Less than 5 years:	120/80
5 to 10 years:	135/85
Adolescent:	140/85 to 145/90

Hyperlipemia

Hyperlipemia (elevated **serum triglycerides** and/or **serum cholesterol**) has been implicated as an important risk factor in the development of CHD, although many researchers attach more importance to **hyper-cholesterolemia** (elevated serum cholesterol alone). Other researchers strongly disagree, reporting that cholesterol is not the villain. (See Monoclonal Cell Proliferation Theory, p. 11.)

Cholesterol is produced by almost all cells of the body (endogenous production), especially by the liver. It is also ingested as a large part of the average American diet. Individual differences in ability to transport and metabolize it lead to an abnormally high serum cholesterol level, which has been purported to result in lipid deposition in the arterial lining. Assuming that low levels are desirable, probably the best way to reduce serum cholesterol is dietary intervention. Although there is some evidence to support the view that regular vigorous exercise is helpful in cholesterol reduction (4, 5, 6, 10), more recent research, using improved experimental design, suggests that exercise effectively reduces only the triglyceride component of blood lipids (7). It is possible that there is a lowering effect specific to some individuals only. However, for the present and until research clearly defines the role of cholesterol in the development of CHD, it seems prudent to maintain levels below 165 and 200 mg% (milligrams of cholesterol per 100 ml of blood) in children and adults, respectively.

It now appears that the manner in which cholesterol is transported might be more important than its serum level. In the blood, cholesterol travels bound to a protein molecule (hence the name *lipoprotein*), either as a **high-density lipoprotein (HDL)** or as a **low-density lipoprotein (LDL)**. A much smaller molecule than LDL, HDL seems to remain suspended in the plasma during its trip through the circulatory system. On returning to the liver, HDL is mostly metabolized and subsequently excreted. In contrast, LDL, being a larger molecule, tends to precipitate and appears to be actively transported into the vascular wall with its protein carrier. It is thought that, as long as the HDL proportion is above 60%, no appreciable lipid deposition occurs.

Epidemiologic research suggests a positive correlation between exercise levels and healthy HDL/LDL ratios, although experimental research has yet to clearly establish it. If this relation does hold, exercise might have a valuable therapeutic effect in the improvement of poor HDL/LDL ratios, in spite of its apparent inability to significantly reduce serum cholesterol levels.

Triglycerides are not ingested directly, as is cholesterol, but are synthesized within the body during carbohydrate metabolism. Although dietary intervention quite effectively keeps the triglyceride level below the 150 mg% recommended by the National Institutes of Health, regular vigorous physical activity has been proven an equally effective method of triglyceride control in some people (7).

Cigarette Smoking

Let it suffice to say that cigarette smoking is one of the most physiologically damaging of human habits, for it plays such a significant role in the long-term development of many degenerative disorders. Smoking only one pack per day is sufficient to increase the risk of myocardial infarction three times over that of a nonsmoker. It is regrettable to view the waste caused by so insignificant and useless an act as cigarette smoking.

Secondary Risk Factors

Of the secondary risk factors, all except sex and positive family history of CHD can be eliminated completely, reduced significantly, or controlled adequately.

Monoclonal Cell Proliferation Theory

Since the early 1970s, a growing body of information has become available that suggests that atherosclerosis might originate from a single mutated cell in the inner layer of an artery wall. This hypothesis, the monoclonal cell proliferation theory, comes largely from the work of Dr. Earl Benditt of the University of Washington Medical School.

Dr. Benditt and coworkers (1), using an electron microscope, have been able to observe the development of an atherosclerotic lesion. They have described its stages as follows:

1   Initially, for reasons unknown, a mutation occurs in a smooth muscle cell of an artery wall (media layer), and the cell divides.

2. The daughter cell migrates into the innermost layer (the intima). This layer is normally populated by only a few cells.

3. For reasons unknown, this daughter cell proliferates and gives rise to a mass of cells, causing a thickening of the intima and eventually resulting in a lumpy plaque.

4. Finally, there is the complication stage, in which a tendency of the cells to degenerate is seen and the lesions composed of more degenerating cells ulcerate.

It is interesting to note that electron microscopy does not support the cholesterol insudation theory, since very little lipid is seen in the early stages of an atherosclerotic lesion (1). The cholesterol that is eventually found in the debris can be traced to one of two sources.

1. Cholesterol can be produced endogenously by the proliferating cells.

2. Cholesterol precipitation from the serum is thought to occur because of an electrical attraction of the cholesterol molecule to ions within the lesion, independent of the level of serum cholesterol (9).

It should be pointed out that this does not necessarily preclude cholesterol from being an important factor in the development of atherosclerosis. For example, it is known that cholesterol epoxide is capable of producing connective-tissue tumors in rats and mice (1). This mutagenic agent is also found in people with high serum cholesterol. Therefore, it is possible that cholesterol has been correctly identified as a villain but for the wrong reasons.

Whatever its explanatory merits, this clone cell theory provides a new framework in which questions regarding the causes of the mutation of the original cell can be pursued.

OTHER HEART DISORDERS

Although the heart disorders that will be described are no less important than those previously mentioned, they occur less frequently and to a great degree are not as preventable as CHD.

Congenital Defects

Congenital defects are abnormalities that are present at birth as a result of some genetic disturbance or developmental problem. Examples are atrial and ventricular septal defects produced by the failure of the heart to make postnatal adaptive changes from fetal circulation to normal circulation, coarctation of the aorta (an obstructive abnormality), and circulatory shunt disorders relating to the failure of certain fetal vessels to close at birth. Although exercise per se cannot remove these defects, psychological outlook and physiologic condition can be improved in those for whom exercise is not contraindicated. Patients with these defects must be handled individually with regard to the level of exercise that can be tolerated.

Valvular Lesions

Abnormalities of the heart valves can (1) occur congenitally, (2) result from some infectious disease, or (3) develop over the years as a result of wear and tear and mineral deposition in the valve leaflets. Some are pathologically significant and some are not. The problems associated with these types of disorders are usually twofold. First, if a valve fails to close properly, there is a backward flow (**regurgitation murmur**) of blood into the chamber from which it came. This produces a volume overload behind the faulty valve and means that the affected chamber has to compensate to keep up. The defective valve is said to be *incompetent*. Second, in obstructive valvular disease, the improper formation or operation of a valve often obstructs flow through the orifice; this problem is termed **stenosis**. In such a case, emptying pressures higher than normal must be generated within the chamber involved. This condition produces a pressure overload in that chamber. The usual result is pathologic enlargement (disproportionate change in the length-width ratio of myocardial cells) of that chamber (hypertrophy). It is not uncommon for a valve to become both incompetent and stenotic.

Initially, these disorders are clinically detected as abnormal heart sounds (*murmurs*) when a physician listens to the heart (auscultation). Since the 1950s, the more serious valvular lesions have been investigated by invasive techniques, such as cardiac catheterization. In this procedure, tiny tubes (catheters) are threaded through veins in the arms or legs and inserted into the chambers of the heart. Pressures in the various heart chambers can then be measured during the different phases of the cardiac cycle, and the degree of valvular incompetence can be evaluated. Use of dyes and X-ray movie photography enables physicians to assess the seriousness of a valvular lesion by observation of a diseased valve and the related blood flow patterns through the heart. Fortunately, many of the more serious problems can be corrected surgically, with the patient returning to an almost normal life-style after a short convalescent period.

In time past, physicians tended to discourage physical activity for people with heart murmurs. Unfortunately, this advice produced an unnecessarily large number of "cardiac cripples." Except in cases of relatively severe mitral or aortic stenosis, in which the risk of sudden death from exercise is high, more enlightened physicians no longer restrict activity levels because of heart murmurs. Instead, they usually encourage each individual to engage in almost any exercise and allow the condition to become self-limiting. In other words, when the circulatory demands of an activity become so severe that the heart cannot pump an adequate amount of blood, fatigue ensues and the individual slows the pace or stops to rest of his or her own accord.

There is no good evidence that exercise can improve the functional ability of an incompetent or stenotic valve. However, exercise-induced bradycardia (decreased heart rate), compensation of the myocardium, and peripheral muscular adaptation are known to reduce cardiac work for a given level of activity. Any adaptation that can decrease cardiac work must be viewed as a beneficial response.

Disorders of Rhythm

Rhythmic disturbances, many of which are relatively harmless, frequently occur in apparently healthy individuals. They are manifest in the form of an unexplained excessively rapid heart rate (tachycardia), extra (ectopic) beats, or skipped beats. Clinical diagnosis can explain some of the abnormalities, but many are transient, occurring in the absence of any pathologic condition, and are therefore inexplicable. (See Chapter 8 for additional information.)

Mild cases of rhythmic dysfunction can be controlled by drug therapy using quinidine, propanolol, or similar medication. More severe disorders require surgical implantation of artificial pacemaker devices.

PREVENTIVE MEASURES IN CHD

The consensus of the medical profession is that CHD can to a great degree be prevented or arrested in most patients but that, once it has progressed to the stage of fibrous plaque formation, the damage is irreversible. In a recent publication (8), one group claims success in reversing the process by means of exercise in combination with a special diet. If further research supports this most recent claim, the current position on irreversibility of the process after plaque formation must be altered.

At the present time, prevention of CHD appears to be a function of early identification of the coronary-prone individual and subsequent control of the risk factors already described in this chapter. Factors that can be controlled, such as high blood pressure, obesity, abnormal blood lipids, high anxiety levels, and excessive sodium intake, must be kept within acceptable limits.

THE ROLE OF EXERCISE IN THE PREVENTION OF CHD

Many claim that vigorous exercise throughout life is a major deterrent to the development of CHD. Another group has claimed that not one case of death from CHD of individuals who habitually trained for and participated in marathons has ever been documented. Whether it is accurate to infer that exercise is responsible for this phenomenon or whether these individuals selected this most strenuous type of physical exercise because of some genetic predisposition is highly controversial. But, at best, it must be said that scientific evidence for justifying such statements at the present time is inconclusive, mainly because of the lack of well-controlled studies using stronger experimental designs than have been employed until now. Even in the absence of overwhelming evidence, and until the evidence becomes conclusive with respect to the benefits of exercise, it seems wise to commit oneself fully to an appropriate physical training program. The limitations and contraindications of such programs are discussed in Chapters 3 and 4.

Finally, the questions of how much one should exercise to prevent CHD and whether, in fact, exercise can prevent CHD are as yet unanswered. Present opinions range from as little as 15 minutes triweekly (for protection) to as much as 6 mi. or 1 hour daily of continuous running at a good pace (to assure complete immunity). Until well-controlled scientific research provides answers, it can be assumed that the benefit derived is generally proportional to the exercise input. This concept is discussed more fully in Chapters 3 and 4.

CARDIAC REHABILITATION

If preventive measures have been begun too late and a cardiac incident occurs, one finds a certain comfort in the knowledge that modern medical technology can in many cases enable a patient to be rehabilitated. Coronary by-pass surgery for reconstructing occluded arteries, valve replacement by open heart surgery, and pacemaker implants are important achievements that have become fairly common during the past decade.

The medical literature is saturated with reports of the therapeutic value of exercise as one mode of rehabilitating patients predisposed to CHD. With few exceptions, cardiac patients respond to physical training in much the same manner as do athletes. In addition to reconditioning the heart, exercise reconditions the skeletal muscles, which some consider to be of equal benefit. Since posttraining heart rate and blood pressure are both lower at comparable work levels, cardiac work is reduced and functional cardiac reserve power is thereby increased (2).

Although many heart attack victims have made remarkable recoveries through rehabilitative efforts involving changes in life-style, the reader should be aware that not all individuals respond well to physical training. Dr. John Cantwell, Codirector of Cardiac Rehabilitation at Georgia Baptist Hospital, has outlined characteristics of a highly trainable postinfarcted patient as follows (3):

1. Less than 55 years old
2. Uncomplicated inferior myocardial infarction
3. Able to achieve greater than 85% of age-predicted maximum heart rate during an exercise test
4. Less than 20% body fat
5. Nonsmoker or ex-smoker
6. Former athlete (physically well-trained individual)

It is interesting to note that half of the items listed are somewhat controllable, and that one (number 6) suggests the value of a physically active adolescence and young adulthood.

REFERENCES

1. Benditt, E. The origin of atherosclerosis. *Scientific American* 236 (2): 74-85, 1977.
2. Bruce, R.A. Principles of exercise testing. In *Exercise testing and exercise training in coronary heart disease.* Edited by J.P. Naughton and H.K. Hellerstein. New York: Academic Press, 1973.
3. Cantwell, J.D. Presentation, Quinton Exercise Stress Testing Seminar, Atlanta, Georgia, January 1978.
4. Fox, S.M., and Haskell, W.L. Physical activity and the prevention of heart disease. *Bulletin of the New York Academy of Medicine,* 2d Series 44: 950, August 1968.

5. Gustafson, A. Effect of training on blood lipids. In *Coronary heart disease and physical fitness.* Edited by O.A. Larsen and R.O. Malmborg. Baltimore: University Park Press, 1971.
6. Joseph, J.J., and Bena, L.L. Cholesterol reduction — a long term intense exercise program. *Journal of Sports Medicine and Physical Fitness* 17(2): 163-68, 1977.
7. Lampman, R.M.; Santinga, J.T.; Bassett, D.R.; Mercer, N.; Block, W.D.; Flora, J.D.; Foss, M.D.; and Thorland, W.G. Effectiveness of unsupervised and supervised high intensity physical training in normalizing serum lipids in men with type IV hyperlipidemia. *Circulation* 57(1): 172-180, 1978.
8. Leonard, J.N.; Hofer, J.L.; and Pritikin, N. *Live longer now.* New York: Grosset and Dunlap, 1974.
9. Passwater, R. *Supernutrition for healthy hearts.* New York: Dial Press, 1977.
10. Pollack, M.J.; Tiffany, J.; Gettmen, L.; Janeway, R.; and Lofland, H.B. Effects of frequency of training on serum lipids, cardiovascular function and body composition. In *Exercise and fitness.* Edited by D.B. Frunks. Chicago: Athletic Institute, 1969.
11. Strong, W.B. The natural history and pathogenesis of atherosclerosis: Pediatric aspects. Presented at the Southeast Regional Meeting of the American College of Sports Medicine, Columbia, South Carolina, November 1975.

KEY TERMS
Asymptomatic (p. 22)
Maximum heart rate range (p. 26)
MET (p. 27)
Stress test (p. 20)
Symptomatic (p. 22)

BEHAVIORAL OBJECTIVES
Upon completion of this chapter, the student should be able to:
1. Define and identify the key terms listed above.
2. Outline the steps to be taken in formulating an exercise prescription.
3. Select and self-administer a suitable test for classification of the functional capacity of the circulorespiratory (CR) system.
4. Describe the precautions that should be followed with respect to beginning an exercise program.
5. Determine a target heart rate for training.

CHAPTER THREE
THE EXERCISE PRESCRIPTION

Although strenuous physical activity is not a panacea for all of the ills of humankind, it is widely accepted that a regular program of vigorous, rhythmic exercise enhances the quality of life by increasing the physical capability for work and play (2). On the basis of the evidence available at the present time, it is not justifiable to conclude that exercise alone is the key to the prevention of heart disease (1), but each year the data become increasingly favorable in support of continued vigorous physical activity throughout life as a valuable adjunct to the elimination of certain risk factors, such as cigarette smoking, high blood pressure, and high blood lipids, in reducing the probability that coronary heart disease will develop.

While it has been established that exercise is, in fact, a valuable tool in the rehabilitation of patients who have certain types of cardiovascular disease (4), and even though the literature supports exercise as a strong contributor to the prevention of atherosclerotic coronary artery disease, caution should be observed before one engages in an unsupervised vigorous program of physical training. Does this mean that exercise is dangerous? Not necessarily. For persons under age 35 who are subject to none of the primary risk factors, the probability of bodily damage from sensible physical exercise is so remote that it can be disregarded. However, there are individuals who could benefit greatly from certain types of exercise regimens at specified tolerance levels but for whom engagement in more strenuous activity might be extremely hazardous or even fatal. There are also a few for whom almost any level of exercise is so dangerous that the risks of mortality far outweigh any small benefits to be gained. These people should not exercise.

The problem, then, is to determine for each individual the amount of risk that is involved, the kind of program that is in order, and the level of exercise that can safely be tolerated. The solution to the problem lies in the analysis of data collected during a procedure designed to evaluate the functional capacity of an individual. This procedure, commonly called a **stress test** or a *graded exercise test*, should be performed prior to participation in any strenuous exercise program.

THE STRESS TEST

A stress test usually consists either of riding a stationary bicycle (bicycle ergometer) or of walking and/or running during a multistage treadmill test while one's blood pressure, electrocardiogram (EKG), and

Figure 3-1. Treadmill stress test.

general response to exercise are monitored by a physician. In either case, the work load is gradually increased in a stepwise fashion until (1) the subject can no longer continue; (2) a predetermined target heart rate is attained; or (3) symptoms of cardiovascular disease are observed, which dictate that the test be terminated. The primary purpose of the test, when directed by a physician, is to identify the presence of silent ischemic heart disease by means of the EKG in the absence of clinical symptoms. Although the testing of persons under age 35 without significant risk factors is not likely to identify more than one case in a hundred, ischemic responses can be expected with greater frequency as age increases (2). In addition to revealing the presence of latent ischemic heart disease, the test is often useful for other reasons (2):

1. To establish a diagnosis of overt or latent heart disease.
2. To evaluate cardiovascular functional capacity as a means of clearing individuals for strenuous work or exercise programs.

3. To evaluate responses to conditioning and/or preventive programs.
4. To increase individual motivation for entering and adhering to exercise programs.

Who Should Have a Stress Test?

Ideally, all who plan to engage in strenuous exercise would be well advised to take a physician-administered stress test first. Even in apparently healthy, **asymptomatic**, young adults, it can be valuable to establish an EKG base line, which can be compared with the results of some future test if the question of an abnormality should arise. Realistically, however, graded exercise tests are quite expensive, and testing sites are often not conveniently located for those who might desire to be tested. Fortunately, people who are able to exercise safely can usually be identified with proper screening during a routine medical examination, including a review of family history of heart disease and a resting EKG. On the basis of the findings of such examinations, the American College of Sports Medicine Committee on Exercise and Stress Testing recommends that candidates for exercise be classified and advised as follows (1):

1. For asymptomatic individuals under age 35 with no previous history of cardiovascular disease, and without any of the CHD primary risk factors, the risk involved in the increase of habitual physical activity is low enough that special medical clearance is not required. If the subject develops questionable symptoms or has not had a medical examination during the previous two years, consultation with a physician seems to be the wise and prudent course before one proceeds with an exercise program.

2. For individuals 35 years or younger who have had or who show evidence of cardiovascular disease or who have significant combinations of positive family history of cardiovascular disease, elevated blood pressure (hypertension), hyperlipemia, diabetes mellitus, cigarette smoking, or obesity, medical clearance is highly recommended prior to any significant increase in physical activity level.

3. Regardless of health status, all persons above age 35 are advised to receive medical clearance before they increase activity levels. Furthermore, it is advised that all persons over age 35 and all those under age 35 who are either high risk or **symptomatic** take an EKG-monitored graded exercise test conducted under the supervision of a qualified physician prior to any major increases in exercise.

Unless one falls into a category that requires a physician-administered stress test, less sophisticated tests that can be self-administered are very helpful in the estimation of one's circulorespiratory fitness level. Two such tests are Cooper's Twelve-Minute Run and the Harvard Step Test. They are described in Laboratory Sessions 5 and 6.

GUIDELINES FOR THE EXERCISE PRESCRIPTION

If the results of a graded exercise test, the presence of certain CHD risk factors, symptoms of cardiac impairment, or age suggest that unsupervised exercise regimens might not be well tolerated, professional guidance should be sought before the individual engages in any activity program. If there are no contraindications to physical activity, it is not hazardous for people to prescribe their own individualized programs. The best results are assured when the exercise regimen is prepared scientifically and is based on the results of a preliminary evaluation of cardiovascular function, on the subject's health, interests, and proficiency, and on available facilities (2). If there has been no physician-administered graded exercise test and there are no contraindications to physical activity, one of the less sophisticated tests described earlier in this chapter should be self-administered.

After functional capacity has been assessed, the first step in the planning of any exercise program is to formulate realistic objectives with regard to the desired kinds and levels of physiologic improvement. Using the results of the preexercise test and keeping the program objectives in mind, the prescriber next chooses:

1. The type of exercise to be engaged in
2. The frequency of the exercise
3. The intensity of the exercise
4. The duration of the exercise

Types of Exercise

The most basic principle behind any type of training is that it should overload the body beyond normal daily demands. Second, training has a specificity effect: only the body part that is overloaded improves, and the improvement is specific to the type of exercise used. Since this is the case, several types of exercise become available for choice. It is important to know the training effect expected from each type. To become physically fit, one needs to devise a program that stresses work in circulorespiratory endurance, muscular endurance, strength, and flexibility.

Circulorespiratory Endurance or Aerobic Exercise

If a training regimen were to contain only one type of exercise, then one that develops circulorespiratory endurance would be preferable. Running, swimming, and cycling are three commonly chosen activities used to develop *aerobic power*. These types of movements, when vigorously engaged in, overload the oxygen-transport system, and an increase in circulorespiratory endurance results. Any activity that involves the large-muscle groups of the body in continuous, rhythmic, *dynamic contraction* is satisfactory.

Muscular Strength and Endurance

It is generally accepted that methods of developing strength and methods of developing endurance lie at opposite ends of a continuum. Strength is best developed by high-resistance, low-repetition exercises that are dynamic in nature. (See Chapter 4.) On the other hand, to improve endurance, either circulorespiratory or muscular, one must alter the traditional strength-training procedure by the addition of further repetitions. If one wants to develop both strength and muscular endurance, the former is usually the initial concern, with high-resistance, low-repetitive exercise being employed until the desired level of strength is achieved. Then the number of repetitions is increased while the resistance is held constant.

Isometric exercise has been proven effective in increasing strength; however, the authors have two serious reservations about recommending this method. First, research indicates that *isometric contraction* appears to enhance strength most at the angle at which contraction is performed. Second, static strains are potentially dangerous to poorly conditioned individuals and persons with reduced cardiac adaptability. At any rate, neither form of strength training is effective in the improvement of the central circulatory function.

Flexibility and Relaxation Activities

As a result of inactivity or aging, the range of motion in joints is progressively decreased. Maintaining flexibility is highly desirable and can be achieved by means of slow stretching movements. A posture at the limit of one's range of motion should be held momentarily, then followed by a further effort to stretch the joint and the corresponding muscle groups. Rapid, forced, ballistic bouncing is not recommended, because tissue damage might occur. It has been suggested that this type of bouncing might even be detrimental to flexibility, due to muscular response to the *stretch reflex*. Additional information on flexibility can be found in Chapter 5.

In recent years, more emphasis has been placed on *relaxation* activities. (See Chapter 7.) Typically, the subject is taught to identify the source of muscular tension. Relaxation is then achieved by vigorous contraction of that particular muscle group while the subject breathes freely, after which the subject makes a conscious attempt at complete muscular relaxation. These exercises are most effectively used during the warm-up and cool-down periods of an exercise session (1).

Frequency, Duration, and Intensity

When planning an exercise program, one does well to remember that the initial improvement in sedentary individuals generally occurs in proportion to the amount of work accomplished. Later, as the physical condition improves, further increases in the work load elicit diminished gains in relation to work input. This necessitates periodic revisions of the exercise prescription if continued improvement is desired. At some point, however, when improvement is no longer the goal, the program changes to one of maintenance. Thus, when one is faced with decisions about how often (frequency), how long (duration), and how hard (intensity), two major criteria should be kept in mind: first, the entry level of the participant and, second, the goals and how soon must they be achieved.

It appears that, except for very deconditioned people, fewer than three workouts per week are not sufficient to produce measurable training benefits. Three per week have been demonstrated to be beneficial for most sedentary persons. After a moderate level of training has been attained, however, the frequency usually must be increased to five workouts per week if continued improvement is to be observed. Therefore, after the initial triweekly period, and except in the case of those who are preparing for world class competition, training frequency should be increased to five weekly sessions interspaced by rest days. These rest days allow the body to rebuild tissues that inevitably become worn and injured, and they offer psychological relief to those who become bored with the regularity of the regimen.

There often arises the question of how the work sessions should be spaced when fewer than five weekly sessions are employed. Participants have traditionally been advised to space training sessions symmetrically on alternate days throughout the week, although good scientific data are not presently available to justify this conclusively. In a recent study involving the placement of triweekly training sessions, researchers found no difference between improvements made by subjects who symmetrically spaced the training and rest days and those made by subjects who worked for three consecutive days and rested for four (3). Despite this evidence of improved aerobic power with nonsymmetrical spacing of training sessions, the effectiveness of exercise in the reduction of serum triglyceride levels for 24 to 36 hours after a vigorous workout appears to make symmetrical spacing advisable.

Intensity and duration are inversely related. For the development of circulorespiratory endurance, it seems more desirable to increase the duration (within reasonable limits) at the expense of intensity, rather than vice versa, particularly in symptomatic individuals over 35 years old. The total exercise period for normal subjects should be about 20 to 30 minutes in length; it should include an initial 5- to 10-minute warm-up period (longer for older and less well conditioned subjects) and should end with approximately 10 minutes of cool-down and relaxation activities. A minimum of 15 minutes of aerobic exercise, exclusive of warm-up and cool-down, is recommended.

Determining the intensity of exercise is probably the most difficult part of an exercise prescription. Several guidelines are helpful, however. It must always be remembered that training effects ensue *only* if the amount of the overload (training stimulus) is greater than some minimal amount of work necessary to maintain normal physiologic function and that the level of this stimulus varies among individuals.

Since commitment to exercise is a lifetime proposition, previously sedentary individuals should not be overly ambitious at the start but should initiate the program at a relatively low intensity and gradually increase the level of exertion over the days and weeks that follow. It should also be understood that the training effect appears to be dependent, at least in part, on the total amount of work accomplished. Therefore, only small gains may be seen in the very early sessions of training in comparison with later sessions of identical length, when intensity can safely be increased. In the early stages, intensities that demand more than 75% of the subject's maximal attainable heart rate are not well tolerated and are therefore not recommended (2). Translated into practical terms, this means that a subject should feel fully rested and not fatigued within approximately one hour after exercise. Otherwise, the exercise program is too severe (1).

Researchers have fairly well defined the threshold necessary to produce measurable gains in function capacity as roughly 60% of one's **maximum heart rate range.** Just as one can train at an intensity too low to be of any benefit (i.e., below 60%), training can also be more rigorous than necessary to accomplish the desired goals. Except in the case of athletes preparing for world class competition, there is no need to train at intensities greater than 85% of one's aerobic capacity. Furthermore, too high a training level might even be hazardous to subjects with exercise limitations.

There are several indices available to quantify the intensity of a training program. It is the wise subject who learns the technique of self-monitoring responses to the training stimulus, both during the workout as well as over the long term. Since heart rate, work load, and oxygen uptake are linearly related in the normal workout ranges, any one of these parameters is suitable for the monitoring of training intensity. Heart rate is the easiest of these to monitor and is probably the most frequently used index: the subject places the first and second fingers lightly on the carotid artery (located in the neck; see Figure 3-2), counts the pulsations for 10 seconds, and multiplies that count by 6 to find the number of beats per minute. Only one carotid should be selected for *palpation*, and the pressure should be very light to prevent stimulation of the *baroreceptors*, which reflexively reduce heart rate. In addition, if an estimate of exercise heart rate is desired, the measurement must be made during the *first* 10 seconds *immediately* after the cessation of the exercise.

The heart rate at which one should work can be calculated very easily, as is demonstrated in the following problem. Assume that an exercise prescription calls for work at 60% of a subject's maximum heart rate range. Assume also that this subject has a maximum heart rate of 200 beats per minute (this is the predicted value for a normal 20-year-old) and a resting heart rate of 70 beats per minute. The effective or maximal heart rate range is calculated by subtracting the resting heart rate from the maximum heart rate, which gives a potential increase of 130 beats per minute. This figure is then multiplied by 0.6 (for a 60% increase), which gives 78 beats per minute. This is added to the resting rate. The target heart rate for satisfying the prescribed intensity level for this subject is therefore 78 + 70 = 148 beats per minute. The resting and maximal heart rate values may change from individual to individual, along with the intensity, but the procedure for calculating does not change. (See Table 3-1.)

An alternative to the use of the heart rate as an index of circulatory stress is gaining wider acceptance among exercise physiologists and medical personnel. This method employs multiples of the resting metabolic rate (**MET**), which represent the amount of oxygen used in the performance of various activities (expressed as milliliters of oxygen

Figure 3-2. Palpation of carotid pulse.

consumed per kilogram of body weight per minute). One MET is approximately 3.5 ml/kg/min. Two METS represent work requiring 7.0 ml/kg/min., three METS represent 10.5 ml/kg/min., and so on.

The maximal functional capacity of most sedentary individuals is about 8 to 10 METS, and, in highly trained athletes, it is about 16 to 20 METS. Accordingly, a work intensity of 4 METS represents 50% of the functional capacity of an individual whose maximum capacity is 8 METS, whereas this same load represents only 25% of the capacity of an athlete whose maximum is 16 METS. Consequently, the intensity represented by a MET is absolute in terms of the amount of oxygen consumed but relative with respect to the functional capacity of an individual. That is to say that 8 METS might be all that one individual can tolerate, but it might tax another individual at only 50%.

Some common activities along with their approximate MET values can be seen in Table 6-9.

TABLE 3-1
DETERMINATION OF TARGET HEART RATE FOR TRAINING

			Sample
1. Predicted maximum heart rate (use actual rate if known)	=	(200)	200
2. Resting heart rate (end of week 1)	= −		−70
3. Maximum heart range	=		130
4. Percentage desired for training (use 60%, 70%, 80%)	= ×		× 0.60
5. Multiply step 3 by step 4	=		78
6. Resting heart rate	= +		+70
7. Target heart rate for training (end of week 1)	=		148

*Periodic revision of target heart rate will become necessary as resting heart rate changes. See Table 3-2.

TABLE 3-2
RECORD OF RESTING HEART RATE

	Resting Heart Rate	Target Heart Rate
End of week 1		
End of week 2		
End of week 3		
End of week 4		
End of week 8		
End of last week		

TABLE 3-3
ESTIMATED MAXIMUM HEART RATE (MHR) BY AGE

Age	15-19	20-24	25-29	30-34	35-39	40-44	45-49	50-54	55-60
MHR	205	200	195	190	185	180	175	170	165

Precautions

In general, apparently healthy, asymptomatic persons whose functional capacities are at least 8 METS can participate safely in an unsupervised conditioning program. For symptomatic individuals, regardless of their functional capacities, or for asymptomatic persons whose functional capacities are less than 8 METS, supervised exercise programs are advised, at least until it is deemed safe for them to exercise on their own (1). Additional precautions seem warranted as follows (2):

1. Exercise should be shunned when it can aggravate a minor illness, injury, or infection or retard recovery from illness. Even when a subject simply does not feel well, exercise could be dangerous, since illness might be incipient.

2. Strenuous exercise is hazardous in unusual environmental conditions (heat and humidity), during times of emotional stress, or immediately after ingestion of a heavy meal. In these cases, the intensity must be decreased or the exercise even abandoned.

3. Cool-down periods should occur in the same environment as the exercise. In no case should one move from a cooler to a warmer environment during a cool-down period after strenuous exercise.

4. Hot showers should be avoided during the immediate postexercise period, particularly in the over-35 age group. In rare instances, hot showers have been associated with immediate occurrence of heart attack.

Summary

In summary, the following steps appear to be reasonable when one makes a commitment to exercise throughout life:

1. Preliminary determination of individual functional capacity in relation to the degree of risk involved in exercise, with subsequent medical clearance or restriction.

2. Development of an appropriate exercise prescription, scientifically based on individual objectives, needs, functional capacity, and interests.

3. Regular, prudent participation in the prescribed regimen, with attention to safety precautions and contraindications to exercise.

4 Periodic reassessment of functional capacity in terms of adaptation to training, with subsequent adjustment of the prescription if indicated.

REFERENCES

1. American College of Sports Medicine. *Guidelines for graded exercise testing and exercise prescription*. Philadelphia: Lea and Febiger, 1975.
2. American Heart Association. *Exercise testing and training of apparently healthy individuals: A handbook for physicians*. New York: American Heart Association, 1972.
3. Moffatt, R.J.; Stamford, B.A.; and Neill, R.D. Placement of tri-weekly training sessions: Importance regarding enhancement of aerobic capacity. *Research Quarterly* 48(3): 583-591, 1977.
4. Naughton, J.P., and Hellerstein, H.K., (eds.). *Exercise testing and exercise training in coronary heart disease*. New York: Academic Press, 1973.

KEY TERMS
Interval training (p. 36)
Jogging (p. 35)
Repetition max (RM) (p. 38)
Set (p. 37)
Specificity effect (p. 34)
Work-relief ratio (p. 36)

BEHAVIORAL OBJECTIVES
Upon completion of this chapter, the student should be able to:
1. Differentiate between types of training programs with regard to expected benefits.
2. Develop an individualized training program for improving circulorespiratory endurance.
3. Develop an individualized training program for improving strength.
4. Describe the procedure used in circuit training.
5. List the physiological adaptations to endurance training.
6. List the physiological adaptations to strength training.

CHAPTER FOUR
TRAINING PROGRAMS AND THEIR EFFECTS

PRINCIPLES OF TRAINING

Van Huss et al. (29) list several goals that are purported to motivate people to train. Some of the more common ones are:

1. Development of physique
2. Improvement of general physical condition
3. Increase in proficiency in sports skills
4. Weight control
5. Rehabilitation from injury or disease
6. Protection from injury

The training procedures used to accomplish these ends take various forms, many of which may not produce the intended outcomes. It is essential that individuals desiring to train understand a few concepts basic to the development of any training program.

First, the **specificity effect** of training, mentioned in Chapter 3, should be emphasized. This means that one benefits only in specific ways from particular kinds of training. For example, if one engages in activities that primarily involve the legs, then the arms do not benefit. Training is even more specific to limbs or muscle groups. Roberts and Alspaugh (28) clearly demonstrated this in an experiment using cycling and running. Thirty-six subjects were tested on a bicycle ergometer and a motor-driven treadmill, after which they were randomly assigned to two different training groups. One group trained by pedaling a stationary bicycle, and the training stimulus for the other group was running on the treadmill. At the end of six weeks of training, each group was retested on both the bike and the treadmill. Interestingly, even though both training procedures involved leg work, the bike group improved only when tested on the bicycle ergometer, but the treadmill group improved on the bike and on the treadmill. From these data, it appears that cycling is a more specific exercise, while running appears to be a more general conditioner. Other experiments comparing arm work and leg work have produced similar results: improvement seems to be restricted to the location of the working muscles (13). Obviously, however, local muscle groups do not improve appreciably without some adaptation of the central circulation to training. Consequently, when dealing with training effects, one must be careful to select stimuli that elicit central circulatory adaptation as well as peripheral adaptation in those muscles doing the work.

Second, the principle of overload (see p. 23) must be reemphasized: without a *stressor* (exercise) greater than that which is habitually encountered, no improvement will occur. The greater the overload, within certain limits, the greater the stimulus imposed.

Third, the training regimen must occur at regular intervals at an intensity greater than a determinable minimal threshold, or no adaptation will occur; once the desired state of training is achieved, continued maintenance must be provided through at least biweekly sessions of the same regimen, or detraining will occur.

As was indicated in Chapter 3, one must decide what kinds of benefits to seek prior to formulation of a training program. It is only after the objectives are clearly identified that decisions regarding exercise type, frequency, and intensity can be made.

TRAINING FOR CIRCULORESPIRATORY ENDURANCE

Circulorespiratory (CR) endurance (also called *aerobic power*) describes a high state of efficiency of the circulatory and respiratory systems in supplying oxygen to the working tissue. Of all of the benefits one might receive from physical training, increased CR endurance is perhaps the most important. There are a multitude of training methods for CR improvement. Two of the most popular are described here.

Continuous Exercise

It has been clearly established that running or jogging long, slow distances (LSD) is an excellent method of improving CR endurance. (**Jogging** describes a slow running pace of about 8 to 12 min./mi.) Depending on the individual's training objective, appropriate distances range from 2 to 6 mi. at an intensity of between 7 and 9 min./mi. Whatever the distance, the pace must be severe enough to elicit a heart rate of at least 60% of the maximum heart rate range, as was described in Chapter 3. Generally, this works out to be about 150 beats per minute for most people 18 to 25 years old.

The importance of the distance-intensity relationship can be clearly seen in the results of a study conducted by the authors, using 20 college-age women enrolled in a foundations class (4). The subjects ran 1.3 mi. per day in symmetrically spaced triweekly sessions for 10 weeks. Although the subjects were aware of the intensity levels necessary to elicit a training response, they were not forced to work at any particular intensity; only the distance was required. A comparison of their treadmill performances before and after the training period revealed no changes in maximum oxygen uptake, heart-rate response to a given submaximal workload, or maximal heart rate. It was concluded that distance alone in the absence of some minimal level of intensity does not guarantee improvements in CR endurance.

Interval Training

In the last decade, a style called **interval training** has been well received as an outstanding method of developing aerobic power. In contrast to the LSD regimen, the interval style of training is discontinuous. A typical interval workout consists of several (three to seven) work periods that are relatively short (usually 3 to 5 minutes each) and very strenuous (approximately 80% of maximum capacity). These are interspaced by rest periods during which the subject walks or jogs while partially recovering for the next work period. The length of the recovery period may be based on a previously set **work-relief ratio** of 1:1, 1:2, or 1:3, or it may be judged sufficient when the heart rate has returned to 120 beats per minute as determined by palpation of the carotid artery.

There appear to be several advantages of interval-style training, compared to continuous work.

1. The intensity of the work can be greater, since the work periods are relatively short.
2. The total amount of work accomplished within a given period of time can be greater.
3. More work can be accomplished with less discomfort.
4. The flexibility of the program helps reduce the boredom of prolonged continuous exercise.
5. The methods available for increasing the work load are more flexible.

The important considerations in the construction of an interval program are:

1. The length of the work period. At least 3 to 5 minutes are required if aerobic power is the objective.
2. The length of the rest period. Acceptable ratios of work to relief are 1:1, 1:2, and in some cases 1:3.
3. The intensity of the work. In most cases, 70% to 80% of maximum capacity is recommended.
4. The number of work periods.

As the individual adapts physiologically to the training stimulus, the work load can be increased by:

1. An increase in the length of the work period
2. A decrease in the length of the rest period
3. An increase in the intensity of the work period
4. An increase in the number of work periods
5. Any combination of the above

Apparently, not all types of exercise are equally effective in improving aerobic power. For example, Fox et al. (18) reported posttraining increases in maximum oxygen uptake when several short sprints served as the training stimulus. The sprinting periods (15 to 30 seconds each) were interspaced with rest periods in the work-relief ratio of 1:3. The authors, using 10 subjects in a similar program, have been unable to replicate these results (5). In another study, Allen et al. (3) used triweekly sessions of circuit weight training to condition 33 college freshmen. During each 27-minute workout, 30-second work bouts were alternated with 60-second rest periods (work-relief ratio of 1:2). Even though heart rates during the entire 27-minute workout far exceeded the generally accepted threshold for the production of cardio-vascular adaptation, no *hemodynamic* improvement was found. The authors concluded that high heart rates alone do not stimulate training benefits but that the type of exercise is important.

The appropriateness of using very short work intervals remains questionable. Reports of increasing aerobic power by means of work periods of less than 2 minutes should be accepted with reservations until a greater body of data supporting these claims can be assembled.

HEMODYNAMIC RESPONSES TO ENDURANCE TRAINING

The training programs previously described in this chapter elicit responses that are specific to the frequency, intensity, duration, and type of exercise engaged in. Furthermore, the changes of adaptation might differ with respect to the physiologic states — rest, submaximal work, and maximal work. The consensus of recent research appears to support the posttraining changes presented in Tables 4-1 and 4-2 and in Figure 4-1.

TRAINING FOR STRENGTH

For many years, the main physiologic benefit ascribed to weight training has been the development of muscular strength. DeLorme (14) wrote that weight training methods can be clearly divided into two types — a high-resistance, low-repetition program for strength development, and a low-resistance, high-repetition program for improvement of muscular endurance. He further suggested that either type is incapable of producing the results obtained by the other.

DeLorme's technique of *progressive resistive exercise*, generally accepted as the standard of weight training during the late 1940s, called for 7 to 10 bouts (**sets**) of repetitive exercise, each set consisting of 10 to 12 repetitions. His patients tried to increase the number of

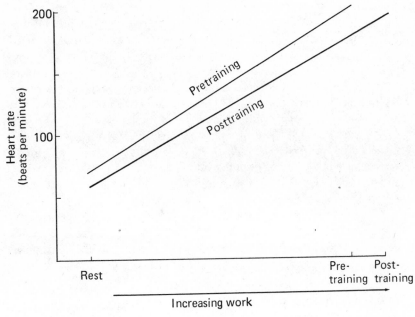

Figure 4-1. Heart rate response to given work loads before and after several weeks of endurance training.

repetitions (**repetition max**, or **RM**) they could execute daily. At the end of each week, a new maximum resistance that could be handled through 10 repetitions (10 RM) was determined. The result was constant overload during the work period.

DeLorme and Watkins (15) later modified DeLorme's original statement on the necessary intensity and duration of the work bout; they recommended that patients (1) begin with only 50% of maximal contraction, to be increased to 100% at least once during the workout, and (2) reduce the 7 to 10 sets to 2 or 3. This procedure was questioned by Zinovieff (30), who advocated reversing the order in which resistance is applied, so that the heaviest loads would be encountered first and reduced systematically thereafter to keep pace with fatigue.

Since the time of these early conceptions of technique, weight training has been studied extensively by several investigators. The consensus appears to support symmetrically spaced triweekly workouts of three sets using the maximum weight the subject can handle for 5 to 6 repetitions; this routine seems to be optimal in producing gains in strength. Research indicates that workouts using heavier loads

TABLE 4-1
HEMODYNAMIC CHANGES AT REST AND DURING SUBMAXIMAL AND MAXIMAL WORK AFTER SEVERAL WEEKS OF CIRCULORESPIRATORY ENDURANCE TRAINING

Parameter	At Rest	During Submaximal Work	During Maximal Work
Heart rate	Decrease	Decrease	No change; slight decrease
Stroke volume	Increase	Increase	Increase
Cardiac output	No change; decrease	No change; decrease*	Increase
Peripheral blood flow	Decrease	Decrease	Increase
Systolic blood pressure	Decrease; no change	Decrease; no change	Decrease; no change
Diastolic blood pressure	Decrease; no change	Decrease; no change	Decrease; no change
Oxygen extraction (ml O_2 per 100 ml blood)	Increase	Increase	Increase
Oxygen uptake (ℓ/min.)	No change	No change; decrease*	Increase

* Slight decrease is due to increased mechanical efficiency.

for fewer than 2 RM or lighter loads for more than 10 RM are not satisfactory alternatives to the 6-RM, three-set combination (8, 9).

Isometric Contraction

A second method used to overload muscles is isometric contraction. Since the work of Hettinger and Muller (21) first appeared in the literature, it has been investigated extensively. Although not without opposition, some research supports isometric contraction as a useful method of devloping muscular strength (7, 10, 19, 24, 25).

Originally, Hettinger and Muller reported that a single daily *static contraction* exceeding one-third of the maximum strength of a muscle and held for a short period is able to produce the maximum rate of strength increase, whereas weekly contractions reduced the rate of gain by one-third (26). The reported rapid increases in strength, with a minimum amount of time involved and with no equipment necessary, have made isometrics attractive. However, of several attempts

TABLE 4-2

PHYSIOLOGIC ADAPTATION OF VARIOUS PARAMETERS
TO SEVERAL WEEKS OF CIRCULORESPIRATORY
ENDURANCE TRAINING

Parameter	Direction of Change
Fibrinolysis	Increase
Hematocrit	Increase
Hemoglobin (total)	Increase
Metabolic enzymes	Increase
Muscle capillarization	No change; increase
Myocardial weight	Increase
Percentage of body fat	Decrease
Red blood cells per mm^3	Increase; decrease*
Serum cholesterol	No change
Serum triglycerides	Decrease
Total blood volume	Increase

* Marathon training.

(11, 12, 20) to reproduce the findings Hettinger and Muller reported in 1953, only one (27) was successful. Since strength appears to increase significantly only at the angle of the contraction, the authors do not consider isometric exercise programs to be effective in the development of strength for activities requiring dynamic contractions. In addition, reports of hypertensive blood-pressure response during isometric work (17) and increased resting diastolic blood pressure after an isometric training regimen appear to contraindicate extensive use of isometrics, especially by those with a compromised heart or impaired arterial walls.

Isokinetic Contraction

A third and relatively new type of strength training is isokinetic exercise. *Isokinetic contraction* unlike isotonic and isometric contraction, maintains a constant resistance to movement and a constant rate of movement, regardless of the changes in force that take place as leverage and mechanical advantage change. It is well known that, after the initial force is applied during many lifts with conventional weights, the ballistic effect reduces the muscle force necessary to complete the movement. At the end of most lifts, *eccentric contraction* must be used to brake the inertia and return the weight to the prelift position.

Although many advocate the eccentric portion as a valuable part of strength development, others believe that the effort used in this type of contraction is wasted since it is not naturally used in most sports activities. Isokinetic exercise, with the help of specially designed devices, eliminates the eccentric portion of the movement and provides for a constant resistance, regardless of changes in the force generated by the contracting muscle. This means that the muscle encounters maximum resistance throughout its range of motion. Some have claimed that the elimination of eccentric contraction by isokinetics results in less muscle soreness.

Steps in Developing a Dynamic Weight Training Regimen

The program that follows is a "cookbook" approach to the formulation of one's own high-resistance, low-repetition program for strength development.

1. The subject must identify the muscle groups in which an increase in strength is desired.
2. Appropriate lifts to stimulate those muscles are selected.
3. The order of lifts is arranged in such a manner that the same muscle groups are not used consecutively.
4. For each lift, the subject determines the maximum amount of weight that can be moved for a set of 5 repetitions. This amount is the subject's 5 RM.
5. The training regimen consists of three sets for each lift. Beginning with the 5 RM, the subject tries to work up to a maximum of 8 repetitions for each lift during each of the first two sets.
6. When the subject is able to accomplish 8 repetitions in each of the first two sets and can exceed 8 repetitions in the third set, the resistance should be increased (at the beginning of the next training session) for that particular exercise until a new 5 RM (step 3) is established.
7. Lifting should occur triweekly on nonconsecutive days.

RESPONSES TO STRENGTH TRAINING

The hemodynamic improvements that occur after several weeks of endurance training are not observed after strength training of equal duration. However, certain *histological* and other biochemical changes are observed in the trained muscles.

1. Muscle fibers increase in size. There are also some reports of increases in the number of muscle fibers, but the evidence is not

convincing. At any rate, this is secondary in importance to individual fiber hypertrophy.

2. Contractile force (strength) and localized endurance increase.
3. Hypertrophy of connecting tendons, ligaments, and supporting bony structures takes place.
4. Articular cartilages become thicker and more compressible.
5. Muscle myoglobin increases.
6. Metabolic enzyme activity increases.

CIRCUIT TRAINING

Circuit training was introduced by Adamson (2) in the late 1950s. This method can be used to improve general body condition, or it can be combined with resistive exercises in a program of circuit weight training for the development of strength or muscular endurance.

The classic circuit program consists of 9 to 12 exercise stations arranged in a circuit. After choosing the amount of work to be performed at each station, the subject is timed during three laps around the circuit (with no rest between exercises or laps). The time recorded is reduced by one-third; the resulting figure is the target time. When the subject successfully completes the three laps within the target time, the amount of work at each station is increased, a new target time is established, and the training resumes.

MUSCLE SORENESS

Engagement in activities different from those to which one is normally accustomed often produces muscular soreness. This phenomenon is observed after both strength work and endurance work. In some cases, pain has been reported to occur during the latter stages of high-intensity exercise. More often, it occurs as many as 24 to 48 hours after the activity. This kind of soreness, which appears several hours after the exercise, causes the most discomfort, since it usually persists for several days.

The pain that accompanies heavy exercise most likely results from the accumulation of metabolic waste products such as *lactic acid.* This pain is transitory and usually subsides shortly after the intensity of the exercise is reduced. Recovery appears to be enhanced by continued, very mild movement. This encourages the removal of metabolic wastes from the affected muscles, since it allows circulation to continue at a relatively higher level than what would be experienced if the exercise were stopped abruptly.

The soreness that occurs 24 to 48 hours after a heavy work bout and persists for several days is less well understood. At least three theories have been advanced in attempts to explain it. Hough (22) has hypothesized that the pain results from structural damage. DeVries (16) has proposed that the soreness results from spasms of localized motor units in the affected muscles. Assmussen (6) and Komi and Buskirk (23) have suggested that overstretching the muscle's elastic components during the eccentric phase of contraction produces the delayed pain.

In a recent study by Abraham (1), the efficacy of each theory was tested experimentally. He reported that the evidence did not appear to support either the spasm or the muscle-damage theory but that the 24- to 48-hour delay can most likely be attributed to alterations in the muscle connective tissue (elastic components). However, the soreness was found to be present in muscles that performed concentric contractions as well as in those that performed eccentric ones.

Recovery from this type of soreness can be enhanced by warm compresses or warm baths, accompanied by light exercise to help prevent adhesions during the healing process.

REFERENCES

1. Abraham, W.M. Factors in delayed muscle soreness. *Medicine and Science in Sports* 9(1): 11-20, 1977.
2. Adamson, G.T. Circuit training. *Ergonomics* 2: 183-186, 1959.
3. Allen, T.E.; Byrd, R.J.; and Smith, D.P. Hemodynamic consequences of circuit weight training. *Research Quarterly* 47: 299-305, 1976.
4. Allen, T.E., and Miller, D.K. The effects of 10 weeks of running at volitional intensity on the cardiovascular systems of college women. *Journal of Physical Education and Recreation*, 49(6): 75-76, 1978.
5. ———. Sprint training for aerobic power. Unpublished report. Wilmington: University of North Carolina.
6. Assmussen, E. Observations on experimental muscle soreness. *Acta Rheumatologica Scandinavica* 1: 109-116, 1956.
7. Berger, R.A. Comparison of static and dynamic strength increases. *Research Quarterly* 33: 329-333, 1962.
8. ———. Effect of varied weight training programs on strength. *Research Quarterly* 33: 168-181, 1962.
9. ———. Optimum repetitions for the development of strength. *Research Quarterly* 33: 334-338, 1962.

10. ——. Comparison between static training and various dynamic training programs. *Research Quarterly* 34: 131-135, 1963.
11. Bonde-Petersen, F. Muscle training by static, concentric, and eccentric contractions. *Acta Physiologica Scandinavica* 48: 406-416, 1960.
12. Bonde-Petersen, F.; Gradual, H.; Hansen, J.W.; and Hvid, N. The effect of varying the number of muscle contractions on dynamic muscle training. *Arbeitsphysiologie* 19: 468-473, 1961.
13. Clausen, J.P.; Trap-Jensen, J.; and Lassen, N.A. The effects of training on the heart rate during arm and leg exercise. *Scandinavian Journal of Clinical and Laboratory Investigation* 26: 295-301, 1970.
14. DeLorme, T.L. Restoration of muscle power by heavy resistance exercise. *Archives of Physical Medicine* 27: 645-667, 1945.
15. DeLorme, T.L., and Watkins, A.L. Techniques of progressive resistance exercise. *Archives of Physical Medicine* 29: 263-273, 1948.
16. deVries, H.A. Quantitative electromyographic investigation of the spasm theory of muscle pain. *American Journal of Physical Medicine* 45: 119-134, 1966.
17. Donald, K.W; Lind, A.R.; McNicol, G.W.; Humphreys, P.W.; Taylor, S.H.; and Staunton, H.P. Cardiovascular responses to sustained (static) contractions. *Physiology of Muscular Exercise*. American Heart Association Monograph No. 15, 15-30, 1967.
18. Fox, E.L.; Bartels, R.L.; Billings, C.E.; Matthews, D.K.; Batson, P.; and Webb, W.M. Intensity and distance of interval training programs and changes in aerobic power. *Medicine and Science in Sports* 5: 18-22, 1973.
19. Gardner, G.W. Specificity of strength changes of the exercised and non-exercised limb following isometric training *Research Quarterly* 34: 529-537, 1963.
20. Hansen, J.W. The training effect of repeated isometric muscle contractions. *Internationale Zeitschrift fur Angewandte Physiologie* 18: 474-477, 1961.
21. Hettinger, T., and Muller, E.A. Muskelleistung and muskeltraining. *Arbeitsphysiologie* 15: 111-126, 1953.
22. Hough, T. Ergographic studies in muscular soreness. *American Journal of Physiology* 7: 76-92, 1902.
23. Komi, P.V., and Buskirk, E.R. The effect of eccentric and concentric muscle activity on tension and electrical activity of human muscle. *Ergonomics* 15: 417-434, 1972.
24. Mathews, D.K., and Kruse, R. Effects of isometric and isotonic exercises on elbow flexor muscle groups. *Research Quarterly* 29: 26-37, 1957.
25. Morehouse, C.A. Development and maintenance of isometric strength of subjects with diverse initial strength. *Research Quarterly* 38: 449-456, 1967.
26. Muller, E.A. Training muscle strength. *Ergonomics* 2: 216-222, 1958.
27. Rarick, G.L., and Larsen, G.L. Observations on frequency and intensity of isometric muscular effort in developing static muscular strength in post-pubescent males. *Research Quarterly* 29: 333-341, 1958.

28. Roberts, J.A., and Alspaugh, J.W. Specificity of training effects resulting from treadmill running and bicycle ergometer riding. *Medicine and Science in Sports* 4: 6-10, 1972.
29. Van Huss, W.D.; Niemeyer, R.K.; Olson, H.W.; and Friedrich, J.A. *Physical activity in modern living.* 2d ed. Englewood Cliffs: Prentice-Hall, 1969.
30. Zinovieff, A.N. Heavy resistance exercises. *British Journal of Physical Medicine* 14: 129-132, 1951.

KEY TERMS
Ballistic stretch (p. 49)
Flexibility (p. 48)
Static stretch (p. 49)
Stretch reflex (p. 49)

BEHAVIORAL OBJECTIVES
Upon completion of this chapter the student should be able to:
1. Define the key terms listed above.
2. Describe six problems and disorders associated with inflexibility and four advantages of good flexibility
3. Determine his or her neck, shoulder, chest, trunk, lower back, hips, and hamstring muscles flexibility.
4. Design an individualized program to develop flexibility.
5. Develop flexibility in joints where there is inflexibility.

CHAPTER FIVE
FLEXIBILITY

Flexibility is the ability of an individual to move the body joints through a maximum range of motion without undue strain. It is not a general factor but is specific to given joints and to particular sports or physical activities. It is more dependent on the soft tissues (ligaments, tendons, and muscles) of a joint than on the bony structure of the joint itself (2). However, the bony structures of certain joints do place limitations on flexibility. Extension of the elbow or the knee illustrates this limitation. Similarly, *hyperextension* of the spinal column is limited by the position and shape of the spinous processes, as bending or abduction is limited by the position and shape of the transverse processes.

Flexibility is also related to body size, sex, age, and activity. Any increase in body fat usually decreases flexibility. Girls are generally more flexible than boys of the same age. From birth to old age, there is a gradual decrease in flexibility as the soft tissues lose their extensibility (4). However, this decrease is usually caused by failure to maintain an active program of movement through a complete range of motion.

Active individuals tend to be more flexible than inactive individuals, as flexibility is predominantly a function of habits of movement. The soft tissues or joints tend to shrink and thus lose extensibility when the muscles are maintained in a shortened position, as happens in sedentary individuals. Habitual postures and chronic heavy work through restricted ranges of motion also can lead to adaptive shortening of muscles. Physical activity with wide ranges of movement helps prevent this loss of extensibility. In summary, flexibility is related to habitual movement patterns for each individual and for each joint, age and sex differences are secondary rather than innate (4).

EFFECTS OF INFLEXIBILITY

Flexibility is an important aspect of physical fitness, and the lack of it can create disorders or functional problems for many individuals. Anyone with a stiff spinal column is at a disadvantage in many physical activities and also fails to get full value from the shock-absorbing arrangement of the spine when walking, running, or jumping. Lack of flexibility in the back can also be responsible for bad posture, compression of peripheral nerves, painful menstruation, and other ailments (4). Short muscles limit work efficiency. They become sore when they perform physical exertion, and, without a good range of movement, the individual is more likely to incur torn ligaments and muscles during activities. In summary, individuals with good flexibility have greater ease of movement, less stiffness of muscles, enhancement of skill, and less chance of injury during movement.

DEVELOPMENT OF FLEXIBILITY

It is impossible to state how much flexibility is desirable, but everyone should strive to prevent loss of flexibility during the aging process. It has been shown that, of the soft tissues, the muscles are most affected by stretching exercises and that both the **static stretch** (a holding position) and the **ballistic stretch** (a bouncing motion) are effective in the development of flexible joints. However, the use of a fast, forceful, bobbing type of stretching induces the **stretch reflex**, which could result in injury to muscle tissue. The amount and rate of the stretch reflex contraction vary directly in proportion to the amount and rate of the movement that causes the stretch. The faster and more forceful the stretch, the faster and more forceful the reflex contraction of the stretched muscle. Static stretching is recommended, as it will not induce the stretch reflex. In addition, it poses less danger of exceeding the extensibility limits of the tissues involved, it requires less expenditure of energy, and it provides greater relief from muscle soreness (1).

Stretching should never proceed to the point of actual pain and subsequent soreness. There will usually be some discomfort, but any aftereffects that do occur should be carefully noted and given time to repair.

Little is known about the minimum requirement for the production of gains in flexibility, but research has shown that improvement is most likely to result from *distributed practice* rather than from *massed practice*. It is better to do sets of stretches for each specific flexibility throughout the day than to do all of them at once. Daily exercise, or at least five days per week, is also recommended. Once the desired flexibility has been attained, three days of exercise per week are probably adequate to maintain the flexibility (2).

The most important specific flexibilities are probably neck and shoulder flexion, back extension, hip flexion, and posterior lower-leg extension (ankle flexion). Hip flexion is performed with the knees straight, to stretch the hamstrings (posterior upper-leg muscles), as tight hamstrings cause an improper pelvic tilt, which is a potential contributor to lower back pain or problems (2).

GUIDELINES FOR DEVELOPMENT OF FLEXIBILITY

The following guidelines are recommended for flexibility programs (2).
1. Practice regularly. Flexibility exercises should be performed several times per day and at least five days per week.
2. Flexibility is highly specific to each joint and activity; therefore, flexibility exercises are highly specific.
3. Stretch gently and gradually to prevent soreness and damage to tissues.
4. The extent of stretching should be gradually and progressively enlarged with full extension, flexion, or both being placed on the joint.
5. Flexibility can accompany strength development if exercises are performed through the full range of joint movement.

MEASUREMENT OF FLEXIBILITY

It should be repeated that flexibility is not a general factor but is specific to each joint. No single test, therefore, can measure the flexibility of all the major joints of the body. The following tests provide an indication of flexibility in various parts of the body.

The shoulder lift test (see Figure 5-1) measures flexibility of the shoulders and the shoulder girdle.
1. Lie prone on the floor. Touch the chin to the floor and extend the arms forward directly in front of the shoulders.
2. Hold a stick or ruler horizontally with both hands. Keep the elbows and wrists straight.
3. Raise the arms upward as far as possible with the chin still touching the floor. Measure the distance in inches from the bottom of the stick or ruler to the floor.

Figure 5-1. Shoulder lift test.

The trunk extension test (see Figure 5-2) measures flexibility of the trunk.

1. Lie prone on the floor with a partner holding the buttocks and legs down.
2. With fingers interlocked behind the neck, raise the chest and head off the floor as far as possible. Measure the distance in inches from the floor to the chin.

Figure 5-2. Trunk extension test.

The sit and reach test (see Figure 5-3) measures flexibility of the trunk and the hips.

1. Sit on the floor with the legs fully extended and the feet flat against a bench turned on its side.
2. While a partner holds the knees straight, bend forward and extend the arms and hands as far as possible.
3. Measure the distance from the fingertips to the edge of the bench. If the fingers do not reach the edge, the distance is expressed as a negative score, and, if they reach beyond the edge, it is expressed as a positive score.

Figure 5-3. Sit and reach test.

TABLE 5-1
FLEXIBILITY CLASSIFICATIONS

	Shoulder Lift (in.)	Trunk Extension (in.)	Sit and Reach (in.)
Men			
Excellent	26 or more	23 or more	7 or more
Good	23-25	20-22	4-6
Average	20-22	18-19	1-3
Below average	19 or less	17 or less	0
Women			
Excellent	25 or more	20 or more	8 or more
Good	21-24	17-19	5-7
Average	18-20	15-16	2-4
Below average	17 or less	14 or less	0-1

SOURCES: C.B. Corbin, et al., *Concepts in physical education,* 2d ed. (Dubuque: William C. Brown, 1974); and R.V. Hockey, *Physical fitness — the pathway to healthful living,* 3d ed. (St. Louis: C.V. Mosby, 1977).

The procedures shown in Figures 5-4 through 5-7 can also be performed to measure flexibility (3).

Figure 5-4. Normal flexibility of the neck allows the chin to move close to the upper chest.

Figure 5-5. Normal flexibility of the hips and lower back allows flexion to about 135° in a young adult.

Figure 5-6. Normal flexibility of the hamstring muscle allows straight-leg lifting to 90°
from a supine position.

Figure 5-7. Normal flexibility of the chest muscles allows the arms to be flexed to 180°
at the shoulders.

EXERCISES TO DEVELOP FLEXIBILITY

The following exercises are designed to develop flexibility throughout
the body. An individual may choose not to perform all the exercises but
only to select ones for certain areas of the body. All the exercises should
have a duration of 20 seconds; they should be repeated three times and
performed on at least three different occasions during the day.

Figure 5-8. Shoulder and pectoral stretch.

1. Stand in a doorway and grasp the doorjamb above the head.
2. Lean forward through the doorway until stretch is felt.
3. Stretch a little farther each time.

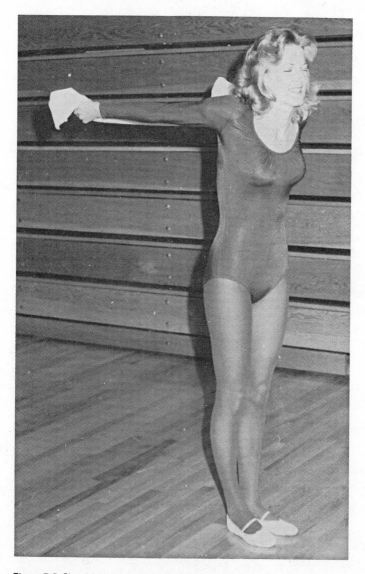

Figure 5-9. Shoulder and pectoral stretch.

1. Stand and hold a towel behind the hips, with the elbows straight and the palms toward the rear.
2. Lift the hands backward as high as possible.
3. Stretch a little farther each time. Do not bend forward.

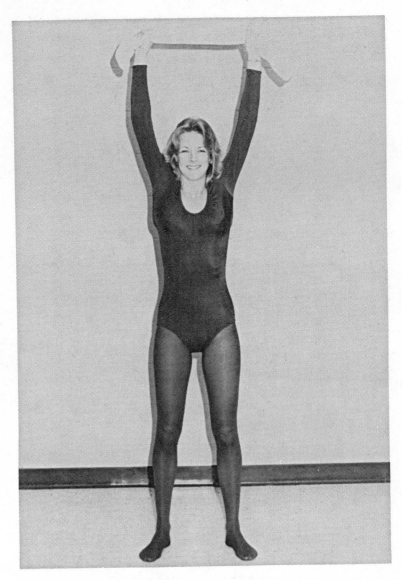

Figure 5-10. Shoulder and pectoral stretch.

1. Stand and hold a towel in front of the body, with the elbows straight and the palms down, about 18 in. apart.
2. Slowly lift the towel forward and overhead.

Figure 5-11. Shoulder stretch.

1. Bring the right hand over the right shoulder to the upper back.
2. Bring the left hand under the left shoulder to the upper back.
3. Hook the fingers of the two hands together and pull.

Figure 5-12. Back extensors stretch.

1. Lie supine with the knees flexed and the feet flat on the floor.
2. Pull in the stomach and bring both knees toward the center.
3. Grasp the knees and pull them toward the chest.

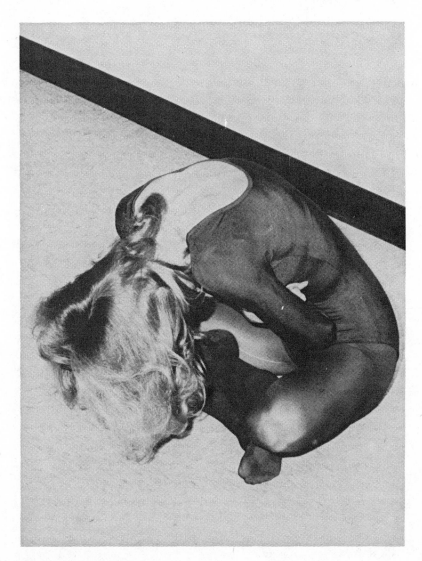

Figure 5-13. Back extensors stretch.

1. Sit with the legs crossed and the arms folded across the chest.
2. Tuck the chin and curl forward. Try to touch the forehead to the knees.

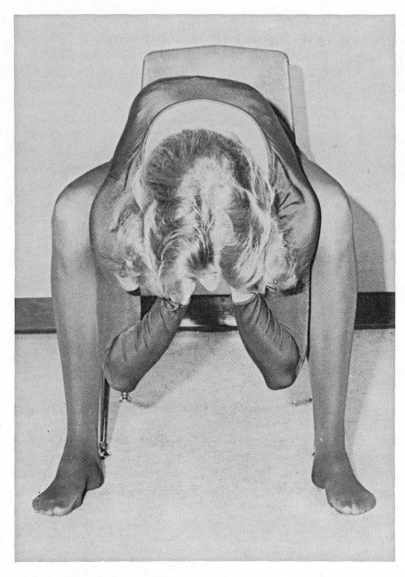

Figure 5-14. Back extensors stretch.

1. Sit in a chair with the feet about 24 in. apart.
2. Bend forward, with the arms and shoulders between the knees.
3. Attempt to touch the elbows to the floor.
4. Stretch until stretch discomfort is felt in the lower back.

Figure 5-15. Upper trunk stretch.

1. Lie prone with the hands in the push-up position.
2. Extend the arms fully to raise the shoulders and upper back. Keep the pelvis and legs on the floor.

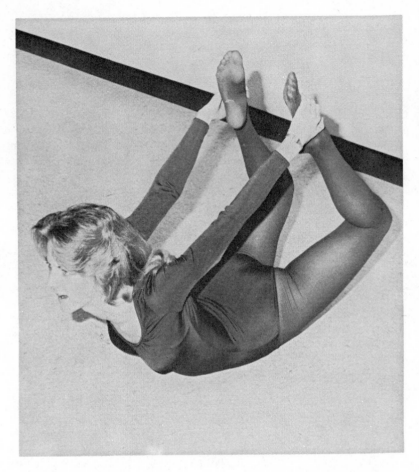

Figure 5-16. Lower trunk stretch.

1. Lie prone, bend the lower legs, and reach back and grasp the ankles.
2. Pull slowly and hold the head up.

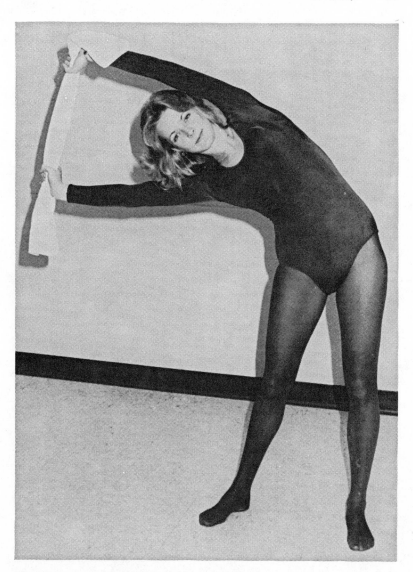

Figure 5-17. Lateral abdominal stretch.

1. Stand and hold a towel overhead with the hands about 12 in. apart, the elbows straight, and the feet 18 to 24 in. apart.
2. Bend to one side as far as possible. Keep the elbows straight.
3. Bend to the other side.

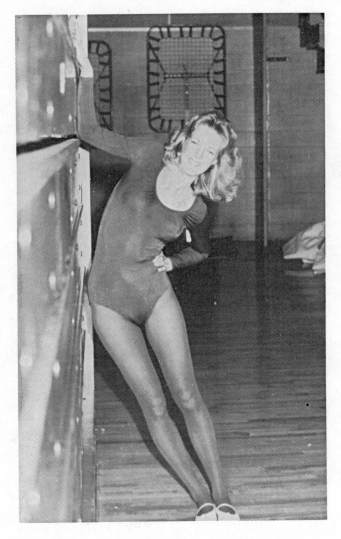

Figure 5-18. Lateral abdominal stretch.

1. Stand with the feet together and the right side toward the wall, about 18 in. from the wall.
2. Place the right hand and forearm against the wall at shoulder level. Place the heel of the left hand on the left hip.
3. Contract the abdominal and gluteal muscles and push with the hand on the hip to move the hips toward the wall. Keep the body straight and facing forward.

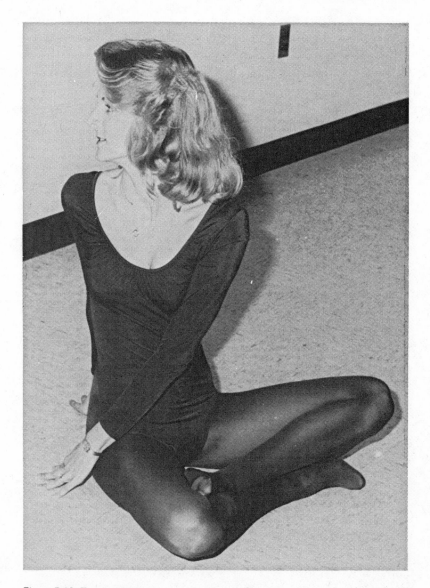

Figure 5-19. Trunk twister.

1. Sit on the floor with the legs crossed.
2. Twist the body to the right and reach to touch the floor behind the back with both hands.
3. Repeat for the left side.

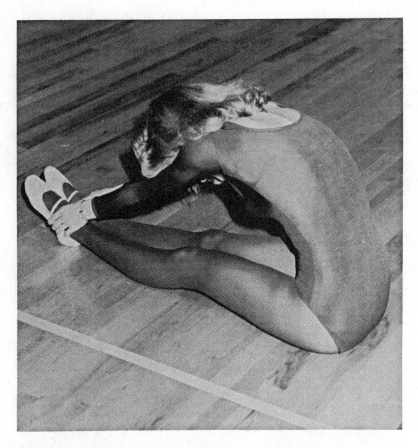

Figure 5-20. Lower back and hamstring stretch.

1. Sit on the floor with the legs straight and the feet together.
2. Bend forward and grasp the outer sides of the legs as far down as possible. Pull the head downward. Attempt to grasp the outer borders of the feet.

Figure 5-21. Hamstring stretch.

1. Stand with one leg crossed in front of the other and with the feet close together. The front leg holds the rear leg back and straight.
2. Slowly bend over and attempt to place the hands on the floor.
3. Repeat with each leg.

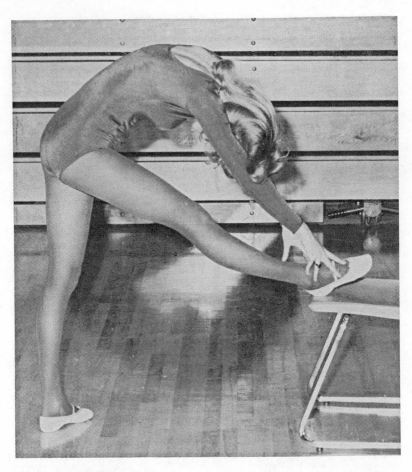

Figure 5-22. Hamstring stretch.

1. Straighten one leg, lock the knee, and place the leg on a footstool.
2. Keep the other leg straight and bring the head to the knee of the extended leg, or toward the knee until stretch discomfort is felt.
3. Repeat with each leg.
4. Progress to the use of a chair and finally a table as improvement takes place.

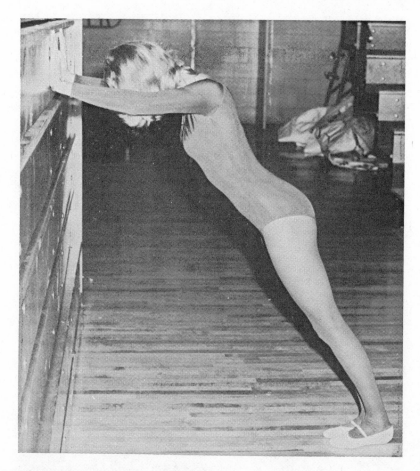

Figure 5-23. Heel cord, gastrocnemius, and soleus stretch (lower leg).

1. Stand with the face to the wall and place the palms against the wall at arm's length and at shoulder height. Keep the feet flat and the body in a straight line.
2. Lean forward and let the elbows bend until stretch discomfort is felt. Do not allow the heels to rise off the floor.

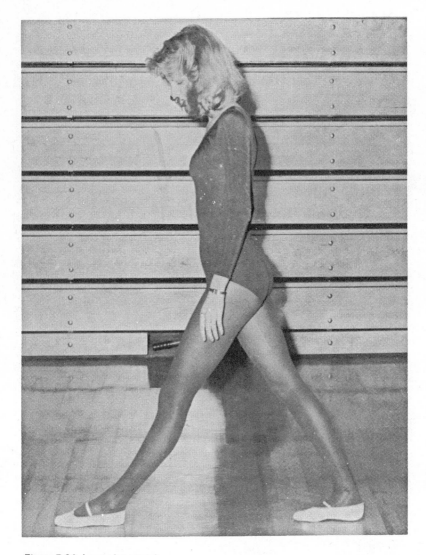

Figure 5-24. Lower leg stretch.

1. Step forward with either leg.
2. Keep the back leg straight with the foot straight ahead and the heel on the floor.
3. Bend the front leg to stretch the back leg until stretch discomfort is felt.
4. Step farther ahead with the front leg to gradually increase the distance between the feet.

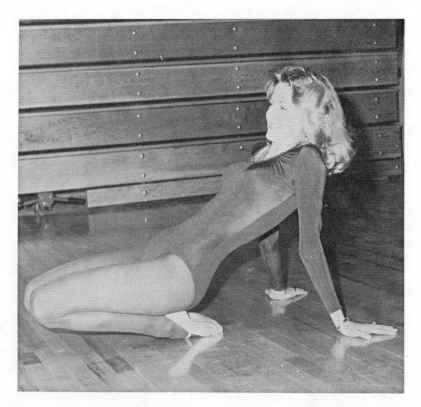

Figure 5-25. Foot and ankle stretch.

1. Sit on the feet with the toes and ankles stretched backward.
2. Balance with both hands on the floor just behind the hips.
3. Raise the knees slightly from the floor.

REFERENCES

1. deVries, H.A. *Physiology of exercise for physical education and athletics*. 2d ed. Dubuque: William C. Brown, 1974.
2. Johnson, P.B.; Updike, W.F.; Schaefer, M.; and Stobberg, D.C. *Sport, exercise and you*. New York: Holt, Rinehardt and Winston, 1975.
3. Neilson, N.P., and Jensen, C.R. *Measurement and statistics in physical education*. Belmont: Wadsworth Publishing, 1972.
4. Rasch, P.J., and Burke, R.K. *Kinesiology and applied anatomy*. 5th ed. Philadelphia: Lea and Febiger, 1974.

KEY TERMS

Adequate diet (p. 76)
Adipose tissue (p. 74)
Basal matabolic rate (BMR) (p. 85)
Calorie (p. 85)
Caloric balance (p. 74)
Hyperlipemia (p. 78)
Negative caloric balance (p. 88)
Obese (p. 74)
Overweight (p. 74)
Positive caloric balance (p. 74)

BEHAVIORAL OBJECTIVES

Upon completion of this chapter the student should be able to:

1. Define the key terms listed above.
2. List the four major reasons why individuals are overweight or obese.
3. List four functions of adipose tissue.
4. Describe five effects of being overweight or obese.
5. Define *saturated* and *unsaturated fat, carbohydrate, protein, mineral,* and *vitamin* and list the functions of each of these substances.
6. Define *cholesterol* and *triglyceride* and list the functions of these substances; state their relations to cardiovascular disease.
7. Describe ectomorph, mesomorph, and endomorph body types.
8. State adequate percentages of carbohydrate, protein, and fat in the diet.
9. Describe a weight reduction plan in relation to caloric intake and exercise.

CHAPTER SIX

NUTRITION AND WEIGHT MANAGEMENT

The way to a man's heart is through his stomach. How often have we all heard this statement? The prevalence of flabby waists indicates that many individuals believe this expression. It is a tragic fact that, even though Americans enjoy the most diverse food supply in the world, a large percentage of them are overweight or obese. Public health records show that 40% to 50% of the population in the United States are **overweight:** their percentage of body fat exceeds a desirable level. One person in every five is **obese,** or has a body fat that exceeds 25% (for men) or 30% (for women) of the total weight (7, 16).

Various causes have been suggested to explain overweight and obesity, but the major reasons are inactivity, overeating, emotional problems, and physiological disturbances. The latter two actually involve only a small percentage of overweight people, and it is these individuals who need medical help. However, inactivity and overeating are without a doubt the major causes of excess weight in this nation's population. These two factors are related, as weight gain occurs if caloric intake exceeds energy expenditure. Inactivity takes on greater significance in combination with modern dietary habits. A physically active man today eats as much as a moderately active man did a century ago, but he is less active than a sedentary man was then (16). Indeed, the single factor most frequently held responsible for the development of excess weight and obesity is lack of exercise (11).

If caloric intake and energy expenditure are equal, there is **caloric balance**, and no weight gain occurs. However, parents often overfeed young children or allow between-meal snacks and sweets while they fail to encourage habits of activity. Later, during the sedentary years of adulthood, creeping obesity occurs because caloric intake exceeds metabolic use or needs, which produces a **positive caloric balance.**

Since so many Americans are overweight, there has been an array of ideas, devices, and diets that guarantee easy methods of weight control or weight reduction, and the public has annually spent millions of dollars in hope that such methods will work. There has also been much publicity concerning the value of special diets and supplements to be used with exercise programs. Unfortunately, most of these methods are not based upon scientific evidence, and their promoters are more interested in money than in the health of the public.

EFFECTS OF EXCESS WEIGHT

Adipose tissue, a type of connective tissue in which many of the cells are filled with fat, is located throughout the body and serves several functions. It is found underneath the skin, where it helps reduce the loss of body heat. It also serves as a reserve food supply, which, if it is needed, can be returned to the cells by the blood and oxidized to produce energy. Adipose tissue is also present around certain internal organs and delicate structures, such as blood vessels and nerves, as protection and support for them; around joints, as padding; and in the marrow of the long bones (10). Obviously, the body needs adipose tissue and should never lack it, but serious problems can develop if there is an accumulation of excess fat. Many individuals only become concerned about their weight because of their physical appearance, but there are other reasons for concern, since there is a direct relationship between fat beneath the skin and internal fat around the body organs.

Life insurance companies have stated that overweight individuals are poorer risks than persons of normal weight, as life expectancy is shorter if there is an excessive percentage of body fat. The death rate is increased 30% for individuals who are 15% to 24% overweight and as much as 80% for individuals who are 35% or more overweight (12).

Diseases of the heart and circulatory system are often associated with obesity. High blood pressure is twice as frequent, and arteriosclerosis (hardening of the arteries) is three times more frequent, in obese individuals (11). For every 5 lb. of excess fat tissue, 4 to 5 additional miles of blood vessels and capillaries must be formed to supply the needed blood. This places an increased burden on the heart and can contribute to the development of cardiovascular disease and diminish the chances of recovery from a heart attack.

In addition, overweight and obese individuals have more problems with their muscles and joints, more lower back problems, and a higher incidence of ruptured intervertebral discs. Excess weight creates respiratory difficulties and increases the probability that varicose veins will develop. Diabetes occurs more often, as do problems during pregnancy, and accidental deaths are more frequent among obese individuals. Being overweight or obese is a threat to the quality and length of one's life.

FUNCTIONS OF FOOD

The term *balanced diet* designates relations among various nutrients in an individual's diet. In the early days of nutritional science, when fewer foods were available, much emphasis was placed on balancing the carbohydrate, fat, and protein in the diet. Research has since shown that the functions of all the nutrients — vitamins, minerals, proteins, fats, carbohydrates, and water — are closely related in cellular metabolism. Hence, the term **adequate diet** rather than *balanced diet*, should probably be used to refer to all these relations.

The best-known and most widely recognized adequate diet consists of groups of foods that provide significant amounts or recommended daily allowances of important nutrients. Foods are grouped into the Basic Four: (1) milk and milk products; (2) meat, fish, and poultry, with nuts and legumes as alternates, (3) fruits and vegetables; and (4) breads and cereals.

There can be a positive or a negative balance of vitamins, minerals, proteins, and the other nutrients, as well as a positive or a negative balance of Calories. It is important that the intake and the needs for all nutrients be balanced (16).

Fats

Fats, or lipids, composed of carbon and hydrogen but containing little oxygen, have the highest energy content of any food. They yield more than twice the number of Calories per gram that carbohydrates and proteins do.

TABLE 6-1
ENERGY SUPPLIED BY THE
THREE BASIC TYPES OF FOOD

Type of Food	Energy (in Cal./g)
Carbohydrates	4.1
Fats	9.3
Proteins	4.1

The body needs moderate deposits of fat for several purposes: (1) to store a reserve fuel supply, which can provide a rich source of energy to replace carbohydrates; (2) to promote satiety or "staying power" during the slow process of digestion; (3) to enhance flavor and palatability; (4) to help provide the fat-soluble vitamins A, D, E, and K; and (5) to support and protect organs (3).

The classification of fats is based on the number of hydrogen atoms combined with carbon atoms. *Saturated fats* are those in which carbon atoms are attached to the maximum number of hydrogen atoms. They harden at room temperature. Saturated animal fats are found in beef, lamb, pork, ham, butter, cream, whole milk, and cheeses made from cream and whole milk. Saturated vegetable fats are found in many solid and hydrogenated shortenings, coconut oil, cocoa butter, and palm oil (used in commercial cookies, pie fillings, and nondairy milk and cream substitutes).

Unsaturated and *polyunsaturated fats* have fewer hydrogen atoms in proportion to carbon atoms. They are usually liquid at room temperature. They are mostly found in vegetable foods and in liquid vegetable oils, such as those derived from corn, cottonseed, safflower, sesame seed, soybean, and sunflower seed (1).

At the turn of the century, the American diet consisted of about 33% fat, but today the proportion has increased to 40% or 45%. Most nutritional experts agree that this percentage should be lowered to no more than 35% and that at least one-half to two-thirds of this total should be unsaturated and polyunsaturated fats. This means that Americans should eat more lean meats, more poultry and fish, and fewer eggs (no more than three or four per week) and that they should use vegetable oils for cooking.

Carbohydrates

Carbohydrates, which make up between 45% and 50% of the American diet, are organic compounds commonly called starches and sugars. These compounds are broken down into a simple sugar, *glucose*, which the body uses as its primary source of energy. Carbohydrates are found in various amounts in grains, vegetables, fruits, and sweets.

Proteins

Proteins are organic compounds that are needed to build and repair body tissues. They make up approximately 10% to 15% of the American diet, but extremely active individuals may require more. Animal meats are excellent sources of protein, but fish, poultry, milk, grains, nuts, and legumes also provide it. The body cells do not ordinarily use protein for energy; they do so only if carbohydrate and fat supplies have been depleted. Protein is especially required during pregnancy. Even though caloric intake should decrease with age, the need for protein does not.

Minerals

The body needs *minerals* in various amounts as building materials for tissues and as body regulators. The more common ones are listed in Table 6-5, but there are others, including chlorine, cobalt, copper, fluorine, manganese, molybdenum, selenium, sulfur, and zinc. Minerals such as sodium and potassium can be lost through exercise, but an adequate diet will replace them without the addition of supplements.

Vitamins

Vitamins do not supply energy to the cells, but they function in the utilization and absorption of other nutrients. They also serve as components of various enzyme systems. They differ greatly in chemical composition. Vitamins are found in various quantities in different foods and must be obtained through the diet.

Vitamins are divided into two groups on the basis of their solubility. The fat-soluble vitamins, A, D, E, and K, are found in foods associated with lipids. They are normally not excreted in the urine but tend to remain stored in the body in moderate quantities. (See Table 6-6.) Due to such reserves, the body is not absolutely dependent on a day-to-day supply. The water-soluble vitamins, B and C, are excreted in small amounts in the urine and are not stored in the body in appreciable quantities (4). (See Table 6-7.)

Some studies have reported various benefits from certain vitamin supplements, and the general public annually spends millions of dollars on these supplements. Perhaps the two most advertised vitamins are C and E. Claims have been made that a vitamin C intake exceeding the minimum required amount can prevent and cure colds, but these studies have been questioned and have not been accepted by all members of the medical profession. It has also been reported that vitamin E can prevent heart disease, reduce the serum cholesterol level, heighten sexual potency, prevent wrinkles, and perform other wonders. However, practically all the miracles claimed for vitamin E can be traced to experiments with tissue damage in vitamin-deficient animals (16). Judgment should be used in taking large doses of these vitamins, and others as well, since they have side effects that can seriously damage the body.

HYPERLIPEMIA

Lipids (fatty materials) that are found in body tissue are also found in blood plasma. If too much of two of these lipids, cholesterol and triglyceride, is present in the blood, the condition is known as **hyperlipemia.** It usually has no outward signs and shows only in a blood test. Numerous studies have indicated that a relation exists between hyperlipemia and coronary heart disease.

The body needs cholesterol for several functions. It is a forerunner of bile salts, steroid hormones, and vitamin D. It also facilitates the absorption of fatty acids from the intestines. However, the body does not depend on dietary sources of cholesterol, because cholesterol is constantly synthesized, mainly by the liver.

There is a relation between the quantity of dietary fat, its composition, and the cholesterol level. A diet rich in saturated fats causes an elevation in the amount of plasma lipids, whereas the substitution of unsaturated fats results in a marked reduction of elevated plasma cholesterol levels (4). Table 6-8 lists the cholesterol level of certain foods. In the United States, there is wide variation in plasma cholesterol levels, but a fasting level between 150 mg% and 200 mg% is considered healthy.

The triglyceride level can be raised by sweets and starches, and it is often high in overweight individuals. The average fasting triglyceride level is 160 mg%.

It is not clearly understood why one individual may have hyperlipemia while another may not, even though both have the same diet.

APPRAISAL OF BODY FAT

There is no simple, objective, and truly accurate method of determining whether one is overweight or obese. Body type, total weight, and percentage of body fat are three criteria used to estimate abnormal body weight.

The morphological classification of body types includes the ectomorph, the mesomorph, and the endomorph (13). An *ectomorph* is a slender person with a small frame: the arms and legs are small, the neck appears long, and there is little definition of muscle tissue. A *mesomorph* is an athletic-looking individual: the shoulders are broad, the hips narrow, and there is a predominance of muscle tissue. An *endomorph* is a thick individual: the arms and legs have a rounded appearance, the chest and waist are about the same size, and the neck is thick.

Three numbers are used to designate the components of each of the three types, with 7 as the highest possible and 1 as the lowest possible rating for each. The first number refers to endomorphic, the second to mesomorphic, and the third to ectomorphic characteristics. The rating 1-1-7 designates a pure ectomorph, 1-7-1 a pure mesomorph, and 7-1-1 a pure endomorph. It is rare to find such extreme ratings; usually there are at least two components of each type present in an individual. A 2-5-4 designation indicates fewer than average endomorphic, more than average mesomorphic, and an average number of ectomorphic, characteristics.

TABLE 6-2
METROPOLITAN LIFE INSURANCE COMPANY TABLE OF
DESIRABLE WEIGHTS (IN POUNDS) FOR MEN AND WOMEN
OF AGES 25 AND OVER (INDOOR CLOTHING)

Height (with shoes on — 1-in. heels)	Small Frame	Medium Frame	Large Frame
	Men		
5 ft. 2 in.	112-120	118-129	126-141
5 ft. 3 in.	115-123	121-133	129-144
5 ft. 4 in.	118-126	124-136	132-148
5 ft. 5 in.	121-129	127-139	135-152
5 ft. 6 in.	124-133	130-143	138-156
5 ft. 7 in.	128-137	134-147	142-161
5 ft. 8 in.	132-141	138-152	147-166
5 ft. 9 in.	136-145	142-156	151-170
5 ft. 10 in.	140-150	146-160	155-174
5 ft. 11 in.	144-154	150-165	159-179
6 ft. 0 in.	148-158	154-170	164-184
6 ft. 1 in.	152-162	158-175	168-189
6 ft. 2 in.	156-167	162-180	173-194
6 ft. 3 in.	160-171	167-185	178-199
6 ft. 4 in.	164-175	172-190	182-204
	Women		
4 ft. 10 in.	92- 98	96-107	104-119
4 ft. 11 in.	94-101	98-110	106-122
5 ft. 0 in.	96-104	101-113	109-125
5 ft. 1 in.	99-107	104-116	112-128
5 ft. 2 in.	102-110	107-119	115-131
5 ft. 3 in.	105-113	110-122	118-134
5 ft. 4 in.	108-116	113-126	121-138
5 ft. 5 in.	111-119	116-130	125-142
5 ft. 6 in.	114-123	120-135	129-146
5 ft. 7 in.	118-127	124-139	133-150
5 ft. 8 in.	122-131	128-143	137-154
5 ft. 9 in.	126-135	132-147	141-158
5 ft. 10 in.	130-140	136-151	145-163
5 ft. 11 in.	134-144	140-155	149-168
6 ft. 0 in.	138-148	144-159	153-173

Courtesy of the Metropolitan Life Insurance Company
NOTE: For those between 18 and 25, subtract 1 lb. for each year under 25.

Body typing can be used to determine ranges of desirable body weight. (See Table 6-2.) A 5-ft.-11-in. endomorph, for example, should not be expected to weight the same as a 5-ft.-11-in. ectomorph. The technique of body typing should be performed by a qualified individual. However, a practical method of estimating one's body frame is to measure the ankle girth at the smallest point above the ankle, with the tape as tight as possible. Compare the measurement with the following standards (8).

	Small Frame	Medium Frame	Large Frame
Men	Less than 8 in. 8'	8-9.25 in.	More than 9.25 in.
Women	Less than 7.5 in.	7.5-8.75 in.	More than 8.75 in.

A modification of the overweight (OW) index (6) by Johnson et al. (9) can also serve as a practical method to determine whether an individual is overweight.

$$\text{OW index} = \frac{45 \times \text{body weight (lb.)}}{2.5 \times \text{height (in.)} - 100} \quad 8\,0$$

Values of 100 or less indicate a satisfactory weight, and values greater than 110 indicate overweight.

Desirable total body weight ranges for certain body types, however, can be mistakenly interpreted if the percentages of fat and muscle tissue are not known. A range from 10% to 15% body fat for men and from 15% to 20% for women is generally acceptable. Individuals with numerous mesomorphic characteristics are sometimes incorrectly considered overweight even though there is a low fat percentage due to the large amount of lean tissue.

Body-fat percentage can be estimated by underwater weighing or by measuring subcutaneous body fat with skinfold calipers. Underwater weighing is the more accurate of the two, but it requires the use of expensive laboratory equipment. Measurement with a skinfold caliper involves pinching a fold of skin between the thumb and forefinger, pulling the fold away from the underlying muscle, and applying the caliper to the fold. The thickness of the fold reflects the percentage of body fat, and therefore muscle tissue should not be included. All measurements should be taken from the right side of the body soon after awakening. Skinfold measurements are usually taken in several of the following areas: over the triceps and biceps muscles, below the shoulder blade, above the crest of the hip, in the chest and abdominal areas, and on the anterior thigh. (Figures 6-I and 6-2 show sites for the measurement of skinfolds in females, and Figures 6-3 and 6-4 show sites in males.) The percentage of body fat can then be estimated through the use of the appropriate formula. (See p. 184.)

Figure 6-1. Posterior surface of arm, mid-triceps.

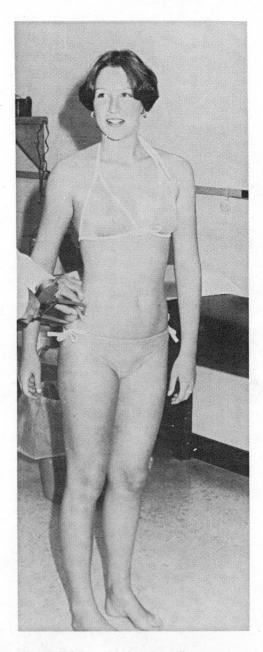

Figure 6-2. Oblique fold just above iliac crest.

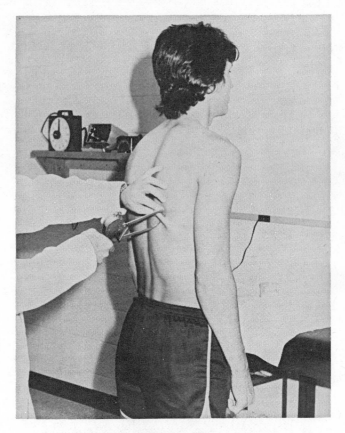

Figure 6-3. Inferior angle of scapula.

Figure 6-4. Anterior surface of mid-thigh.

CALORIE NEEDS

A **Calorie**, or kilocalorie, is the measurement of a unit of energy and is defined as the amount of heat required to raise the temperature of 1 kg (2.2 lb.) of water 1° C. The energy value of food is expressed in Calories.

Calories are involved in all chemical reactions in the body. These reactions, referred to as *metabolism*, include processes in which food is broken down so that energy is released and those in which new substances are produced to store energy within the body.

A considerable amount of energy must be used to maintain certain vital functions — respiration, heart contraction, glandular secretions. This release of energy is called **basal metabolic rate (BMR)** and is measured when the individual is awake, reclined, and relaxed. The number of Calories required for basal metabolism varies with the age, weight, stature, hormone production, and sex of the individual, with females needing fewer than males.

Normal basal metabolism burns about 1 Calorie per hour for each kilogram of body weight. The number of Calories that a man requires per day can be estimated to be his weight in pounds multiplied by 11; 1320 multiply by 10 for a woman, whose BMR is about 10% lower than a man's (5). The average adult male needs approximately 1400 to 1800 Cal./day for his basal metabolism, whereas the average adult female needs approximately 1200 to 1400. Table 6-3 presents the suggested basal metabolic rates for adults.

In proportion to body weight, BMR is highest during childhood and gradually diminishes throughout life. The decline begins during late adolescence, and the slope takes form at about the age of 25 in men and a little earlier, at about 22, for women. With increasing age, there is a gradual reduction in the number and size of functional cells, and muscle cells become fewer and are replaced by fat cells. The rate of decline in BMR is usually between 5% and 7% for each decade of life (5).

The amount of energy needed to perform functions other than basal metabolism varies in relation to daily activities. An extremely inactive individual may need only a few hundred additional Calories, whereas a large, active man may need as many as 2000 or more. Table 6-4 shows the number of Calories needed in addition to BMR.

Individuals generally become less active during the aging process. This reduction of activity together with the decline in BMR indicates that eating habits should be adjusted as one grows older, to prevent gains in weight or increases in body-fat percentage. Consider Mr. Jones, whose case is based on experimental fact (5).

TABLE 6-3
SUGGESTED BASAL METABOLIC RATES
FOR ADULTS

Height (in in. and in cm)		Weight (in lb. and in kg)		BMR (in Cal./day)
		Men		
60	152			
62	158			
64	163	133 ± 11	60 ± 5	1630
66	168	142 ± 12	64 ± 5	1690
68	173	151 ± 14	69 ± 6	1775
70	178	159 ± 14	72 ± 6	1815
72	183	167 ± 15	76 ± 7	1870
74	188	175 ± 15	80 ± 7	1933
76	193	182 ± 16	83 ± 7	1983
		Women		
60	152	109 ± 9	50 ± 4	1399
62	158	115 ± 9	52 ± 4	1429
64	163	122 ± 10	56 ± 5	1487
66	168	129 ± 10	59 ± 5	1530
68	173	136 ± 10	62 ± 5	1572
70	178	144 ± 11	66 ± 5	1626
72	183	152 ± 12	69 ± 5	1666

Adapted with permission of the National Academy of Sciences

TABLE 6-4
ENERGY NEED IN ADDITION TO BMR

Activity	Energy Need (in Cal. per kg of body weight)	
	Men	*Women*
Very light	1.5	1.3
Light	2.9	2.6
Moderate	4.3	4.1
Heavy	8.4	8.0

Adapted with permission of the National Academy of Sciences

When he leaves college, at 22, he weighs 160 lb. He is not a letter-winning athlete, but he is physically active. About 12% of his weight, or just under 20 lb., is fat. Look at Jones 35 years later, at the age of 57. He is proud that he weighs no more than he did when he graduated. However, he rarely exercises and has failed to maintain a regular exercise program since graduation. His body composition is radically different: he has fewer muscle cells and more fat cells. Instead of 12% fat, he now has 24%, or some 40 lb.

And what if Jones had followed a more characteristic pattern? Suppose he had gained 20 lb. in those 35 years, a rate of only about 9 oz. per year. Those 20 lb. would be fat, so that Jones would now have about 60 lb. of fat, out of a total weight of 180 lb.: he would be one-third fat. A very slight modification in eating habits or a regular exercise program would have prevented this accumulation.

It is difficult to determine how many Calories are required to maintain a constant weight. Perhaps the best method is to keep a record of what is eaten for a week during which no weight gain or loss occurs; then calculate the number of Calories (Table 6-8) and divide by 7 to determine the average daily caloric intake. Compare the result with the following estimate: a moderately active adult whose weight is constant consumes the number of Calories approximately equal to 15 times his weight in pounds.

Weight Reduction

There is no quick and easy method to reduce body weight. Extreme low-caloric diets can result in rapid weight loss, but usually an individual will return to former eating habits and regain what was lost. Diets that emphasize excessive consumption of certain foods and elimination of others often result in poor nutrition and can cause more damage than the excess weight.

Guidelines

There are certain guidelines that, if followed, should help the individual in a weight-reduction plan.

1. The body needs all types of nutrients, and the diet should consist of a variety of sources that includes all of them. One of the dangers of Calorie counting for weight reduction is that it may lead to an inadequate intake of certain nutrients. Unless one is advised differently by a physician, the diet should consist of 40% to 50% carbohydrates, 10% to 20% protein, and 30% to 35% fat. At least one-half to two-thirds of the total fat should be unsaturated.

2. A reducing program should include a decrease in caloric intake and an exercise program. By combining these two factors, the individual does not have to cut down the caloric intake as much; the loss of fat is greater, and there is an increase in the percentage of lean tissue. If the loss of weight is accomplished strictly by means of diet, there is a loss of lean tissue as well as fat (17).

3. Weight will be lost only if there is a **negative caloric balance** (use exceeds intake). If there is a positive caloric balance (intake exceeds use), there will be a weight gain. The body stores excess Calories, whatever the source, in the form of fat.

4. The weight reduction should be a gradual one, with a loss of no more than 1 or 2 lb. per week.

5. There should be an attempt to base the amount of weight reduction on the percentage of excess body fat. However, it is difficult to determine body fat without professional help, and therefore the percentage may have to be estimated.

6. Heavy meals should be avoided. Determine the total number of Calories per day the diet will permit and divide by the number of meals. If a between-meal snack is desired, subtract the Calories it provides from the total number before dividing. For example, suppose that an individual who is on a diet of 2000 Cal./day eats a daily 200-Cal. snack. This leaves 1800 Cal. for three meals, or 600 Cal. each; the individual might divide it into portions of 500, 800, and 500 Cal. without a heavy meal.

7. Dehydration or extreme water loss should be avoided. At the beginning of an exercise program, there may be a rapid initial weight reduction due to water loss, but the body will correct this water imbalance within a few days. If thirst is experienced, there should be an intake of water.

8. Attempts at spot reducing are not very effective. The public has spent much money on devices designed for such programs, when general exercise programs would have been better.

9. If the reduced caloric intake is constant, the rate of weight loss will decrease as time increases, due to a smaller difference between total caloric demand of the body and intake.

10. If two people are on the same caloric diet, the heavier or taller person will lose weight faster, due to a higher basal metabolic rate.

11. If a male and a female of the same age, weight, etc. are on the same caloric diet, the male will lose weight faster than the female, due to a higher basal metabolic rate.

Diet and Exercise

Two fallacies concerning diet and exercise often mislead the public. One is that exercise always increases the appetite and therefore results in no weight loss. The other is that exercise expends only a small number of Calories and hence only an exhaustive program can be beneficial.

The facts are, first, that an overweight individual who begins an exercise program usually makes better use of food intake and utilizes stored fat for energy. An underweight individual or one whose weight is correct usually has an increase in appetite as a result of exercise.

Second, the expenditure of Calories through exercise is cumulative. If 250 Cal. were used each day for exercise, 1750 would be used during a week's period. Since approximately 3500 Cal. equal 1 lb. of body fat, this would result in the loss of 0.5 lb. of body fat per week, if everything else remains equal, or 26 lb. in a year. The following example is for a 145-lb. female who wishes to lose 20 lb.

Previous daily caloric intake	2800
Calories deducted from diet	300
Calories used in exercise	200
Daily caloric deficit	500

$$20 \text{ lb.} \times 3500 \text{ Cal./lb.} = 70{,}000 \text{ Cal.}$$
$$70{,}000 \text{ Cal.} \div 500 \text{ deficit Cal./day} = 140 \text{ days} = 20 \text{ weeks}$$

This program takes 20 weeks to produce a loss of 20 lb. It may actually require more days, due to the decreasing difference between total caloric demand and intake as weight is lost.

This rate of loss may appear slow to some individuals, but it is a sensible program. It does not require starvation or extremely hard exercise. Abstaining from one 10-oz. soft drink and one average slice of pound cake amounts to avoiding the intake of 310 Cal. (Table 6-8). Many desserts amount to more than 200 Cal. If this female were to ride a bicycle for 60 minutes at 5 mph, she would expend 217 Cal. (Table 6-9). Furthermore, this bicycle riding would not have to be done in 60 continuous minutes for this amount of caloric expenditure to take place; it could be done several times throughout the day if the total time amounted to 60 minutes. Walking for 45 minutes is another light exercise that would expend more than 200 Cal. for this female. The reader should realize from this illustration and through the use of Tables 6-8 and 6-9 that a daily caloric deficit of 500 Cal. is not an unrealistic goal.

TABLE 6-5
MINERAL SOURCES, FUNCTIONS, ADULT REQUIREMENTS, AND DEFICIENCY DISORDERS

Mineral	Sources	Functions	Adult Requirement	Deficiency Disorders
Calcium	Milk, most dairy products, shellfish, egg yolk, green vegetables	Major component of skeleton & teeth; essential for clotting of blood, normal functioning of nerve tissue	800 mg	Rickets (principal cause is deficiency of vitamin D), demineralization of bone
Iodine	Seafoods, vegetables grown on iodine-rich soils, iodized salt	Formation of thyroid hormone	0.15-0.30 mg	Goiter
Iron	Liver, lean meats, shellfish, egg yolk, dried fruits, nuts, green leafy vegetables	Oxygen transport & cellular respiration	10-15 mg	Anemia
Magnesium	Almonds, lima beans, peanuts, peas, pecans, brown rice, whole wheat, walnuts	Activation of many of body's enzymes; cardiac & skeletal muscles & nervous tissue depend on a proper balance between calcium & magnesium	300 mg	True dietary deficiency has not been reported; it can result from severe renal disease, hepatic cirrhosis, sustained losses of gastrointestinal secretions

TABLE 6-5, CONTINUED

Mineral	Sources	Functions	Adult Requirement	Deficiency Disorders
Phosphorus	Milk, fish, poultry, eggs	Important role in muscle energy metabolism; carbo-hydrate, protein, & fat metabo-lism; nervous-tissue metabolism; normal blood chemistry; skeletal growth; tooth development; transport of fatty acids	800 mg	Deficiency rarely found; abnormal ratio of calcium & phosphorus interferes with absorp-tion of both elements
Potassium	Bananas, beets, molasses, sweet potatoes, green vegetables	Influence on contractility of smooth, skeletal, & cardiac muscle; affects excitability of nerve tissue	. . . . . .	Deficiency rarely found, but it can cause muscular weakness & nervous irritability
Sodium	Celery, beet greens, kale, sodium chloride	Important in acid/base balance & osmotic pressure of extracellular fluids	2.5 g	Muscular cramps, weakness, headache, interference with heat-regulating power of body

TABLE 6-6

FAT-SOLUBLE VITAMIN SOURCES, FUNCTIONS, ADULT REQUIREMENTS, AND DEFICIENCY DISORDERS

Vitamin	Sources	Functions	Requirement	Deficiency Disorders
A	Liver, eggs, fishliver oils; as carotene (converted to vitamin A) in dark green & deep yellow vegetables & yellow fruits	Normal growth of epithelial tissues, normal vision, growth of bones & teeth	5,000 IU	Night blindness; rough, unhealthy skin
D	Salmon, sardines, fish, butter & cream products, liver oils, egg yolk, sunlight; artificial enrichment of suitable foods	Increase in utilization & retention of calcium & phosphorus, which ensures conditions favorable to normal mineralization of growing bone	400 IU	Inadequate intestinal absorption of calcium & phosphorus, demineralization of bone
E	Cereal seed oils, soybean oil, wheat germ oil, green leafy vegetables, legumes, nuts	Prevention of unwanted oxidation of polyunsaturated fatty acids & fat-soluble compounds	30 IU	Deficiencies rarely reported
K	Green leafy vegetables; most important source is intestinal bacterial flora, which provide adequate amount under normal circumstances	Synthesis of prothrombin by liver (blood-clotting mechanism)	Unknown	Deficiency rarely found

TABLE 6-7

WATER-SOLUBLE VITAMIN SOURCES, FUNCTIONS, ADULT REQUIREMENTS, AND DEFICIENCY DISORDERS

Vitamin	Sources	Functions	Adult Requirement	Deficiency Disorders
B_1 (thiamine)	Lean meats, eggs, whole grain products, green leafy vegetables, nuts, legumes	Carbohydrate metabolism, nerve function	0.4 mg per 1000 Cal.	Beriberi, neuritis
B_2 (riboflavin)	Milk, cheese, meats, eggs, green leafy vegetables, whole grains, legumes	Catalysis in cellular oxidations	0.6 mg per 1000 Cal.	Fissures at angles of mouth, inflammation of tongue, visual fatigue
Niacin	Liver, meats, fish, whole grains, bread, cereals, dried peas & beans, nuts, peanut butter	Promotion of growth; important in utilization of all major nutrients	6.6 mg per 1000 Cal.	Pellagra (skin disease), nervous disorders
B_6	Liver, cereals, fish, vegetables	Protein metabolism, cell function	2 mg	Nerve inflammation, skin irritations
B_{12}	Food of animal origin, fish, milk	Formation of blood; fat & sugar metabolism; promotion of growth	3 μg	Pernicious anemia, neuritis
C (ascorbic acid)	Citrus fruits and their juices, potatoes, peppers, cabbage, tomatoes, broccoli	Metabolism of amino acids, healing of wounds, structural integrity of capillary walls, formation of intercellular substance of collagenous and fibrous tissue	50-100 mg	Scurvy, delayed healing of wounds, spongy gums, hemorrhages

TABLE 6-8
CALORIC AND CHOLESTEROL VALUES OF CERTAIN FOODS

Food	Serving	Cal.	Cholesterol
Vegetables			
Asparagus	10 stalks	25	N
Beans, baked	1 C.	200	N
Beans, lima	1 C.	150	N
Beans, green	1 C.	25	N
Beets	1 C.	75	N
Broccoli	1 C.	45	N
Cabbage, cooked	1 C.	45	N
Carrots, cooked	1 C.	50	N
Celery	1 stalk	15	N
Corn	1 ear	100	N
Lettuce	1 head	50	N
Mushrooms	1 C.	30	N
Peas, cooked	1 C.	110	N
Potatoes, baked	1 med.	125	N
Potato chips	10 med.	100	N
Potatoes, french fried	6	100	M
Spinach, boiled	1 C.	100	N
Squash	1 C.	35	N
Tomato	1 med.	25	N
Turnips	1 C.	45	N
Yams, baked	1 ave.	200	N
Animal Meats			
Bacon	2 strips	75	L
Beef, ground	4 oz.	410	H
Beef, pot roast	4 oz.	250	H
Beef, roast	4 oz.	200	H
Beef, steak	4 oz.	200	H
Ham	1 sl.	100	H

NOTE: The following abbreviations are used:

ave. = average	med. = medium	sl. = slice	sq. = square
C = cup	oz. = ounce	sm. = small	T. = tablespoon
lg. = large			

The following symbols are used to represent cholesterol levels:

H = high   L = low
M = medium   N = none

TABLE 6-8, CONTINUED

Food	Serving	Cal.	Cholesterol
Ham, smoked	4 oz.	450	H
Liver, beef	4 oz.	150	H
Liver, calf	4 oz.	160	H
Sausage	1 link	75	H
Veal chop	4 oz.	150	L
Veal cutlet	4 oz.	125	L
Veal roast	4 oz.	250	L
Veal steak	4 oz.	250	L
Chicken			
Broiled	½ med.	200	L
Fried	½ med.	325	M
Livers	4 oz.	150	H
Pot pie	4 oz.	350	M
Salad	4 oz.	225	L
Turkey			
Baked	4 oz.	250	L
Hash	4 oz.	175	L
Soups			
Beef broth	1 C.	35	L
Bean	1 C.	225	L
Chicken	1 C.	100	L
Chili	1 C.	350	M
Tomato	1 C.	100	N
Vegetable	1 C.	100	N
Beverages			
Beer	8 oz.	175	N
Cider	1 C.	100	N
Coffee, black	1 C.	0	N
Grapefruit juice	6 oz.	75	N
Ice cream soda	1	350	M
Milk, chocolate	1 C.	225	H
Orange juice	6 oz.	75	N
Pineapple juice	6 oz.	95	N

TABLE 6-8, CONTINUED

Food	Serving	Cal.	Cholesterol
Soft drinks	10 oz.	120	N
Tea, black	1 C.	0	N
Tomato juice	6 oz.	50	N

Dairy Products

Food	Serving	Cal.	Cholesterol
American cheese	1 oz.	105	H
Butter	1 T.	100	H
Cheddar cheese	1 oz.	105	H
Cottage cheese	½ C.	105	L
Cream	1 T.	50	H
Egg, boiled	1 med.	70	H
Egg, fried	1 med.	100	H
Egg, scrambled	1 med.	135	H
Milk, dried skim	1 T.	25	L
Milk, evaporated	1 C.	200	H
Milk, skim	1 C.	85	L
Milk, whole	1 C.	170	H
Yogurt, skim	1 C.	115	L

Seafood

Food	Serving	Cal.	Cholesterol
Clams, steamed	12	100	L
Clams, fried	2	200	L
Flounder, fried	4 oz.	150	L
Flounder, raw	4 oz.	78	L
Lobster	½ C.	65	M
Lobster Newburg	ave.	350	H
Oysters, fried	6 med.	240	H
Salmon, broiled	4 oz.	140	L
Salmon, canned	½ C.	200	L
Scallops	4 oz.	90	L
Shrimp	10 med.	100	M
Shrimp creole	ave.	175	M
Shrimp, fried	10 med.	315	H
Tuna, canned	3 oz.	170	L

Breads and Cereals

Food	Serving	Cal.	Cholesterol
Biscuits, baking powder	1 lg.	55	L
Biscuits, buttermilk	1 lg.	110	L

TABLE 6-8, CONTINUED

Food	Serving	Cal.	Cholesterol
Bread, cinnamon	1 sl.	200	L
Bread, french	1 sl.	50	L
Bread, protein	1 sl.	40	L
Bread, raisin	1 sl.	75	N
Bread, white	1 sl.	65	N
Bread, whole wheat	1 sl.	65	N
English muffin	1 ave.	150	L
Muffin	1 sm.	125	M
Pancake	1 sm.	100	M
Rice, brown	1 C.	130	N
Rice, converted	1 C.	130	N
Rice, white	1 C.	200	N
Rolls, cinnamon	1 ave.	100	M
Rolls, hot dog	1	125	N
Rolls, plain	1	100	N
Waffle	1	225	M
Fresh Fruits*			
Apple	1 sm.	75	N
Banana	1 med.	100	N
Blueberries	1 C.	80	N
Cantaloupe	½ med.	40	N
Cherries, unpitted	1 C.	95	N
Grapefruit	½ sm.	50	N
Grapes	1 C.	90	N
Orange	1 med.	75	N
Peach	1 ave.	45	N
Pear	1 ave.	95	N
Pineapple	1 C.	75	N
Strawberries	1 C.	55	N
Watermelon	1 med.	100	N
Candies and Nuts			
Almonds	12	100	N
Caramel	1 med.	75	M
Chocolate bar	1 sm.	300	H
Fudge	1 sq.	110	L

*Frozen fruits have additional calories.

TABLE 6-8, CONTINUED

Food	Serving	Cal.	Cholesterol
Peanuts	10	100	N
Peanut butter	1 T.	100	N
Pecans	8	50	N
Popcorn, butter	1 C.	150	M
Walnuts	4	100	N
Desserts			
Cookies, brownies	1 sq.	50	H
Cookies, butter	6 sm.	100	H
Cookies, chocolate chip	3 sm.	65	M
Cookies, oatmeal	2 sm.	50	M
Cookies, vanilla wafers	3 sm.	50	L
Cake, angel food	ave.	100	N
Cake, cheese	1 sm.	350	H
Cake, chocolate	ave.	250	H
Cake, pound	ave.	200	H
Danish pastry	ave.	200	H
Doughnut	ave.	150	H
Eclair	ave.	275	H
Fruitcake	1 sm.	250	L
Gelatin, sweet	ave.	100	N
Ice cream	1 scoop	150	M
Ice milk	1 scoop	100	L
Pie, 1 crust	ave.	250	M
Pie, 2 crusts	ave.	350	M
Sherbet	1 scoop	100	L
Sundae, fancy	ave.	400	H
Potpourri			
Catsup	1 T.	25	N
Cranberry sauce	3 T.	100	N
Honey	1 T.	65	N
Jam or jelly	1 T.	50	N
Maple syrup	1 T.	60	N
Mayonnaise	1 T.	100	M
Molasses	1 T.	50	N
Mustard	1 T.	10	N
Pickles, dill	ave.	15	N
Salad dressing, french	1 T.	100	L

TABLE 6-9

ENERGY EXPENDITURE FOR VARIOUS PHYSICAL ACTIVITIES

Activity	Cal./lb.			METS*
	1 Min.	*15 Min.*	*30 Min.*	
Archery	0.0342	0.513	1.026	4.38
Basketball	0.0530	0.795	1.590	6.80
Bicycling (level road)				
5 mph	0.0250	0.375	0.750	3.21
10 mph	0.0500	0.750	1.500	6.41
13 mph	0.0720	1.080	2.160	9.23
Bowling	0.0486	0.729	1.458	6.23
Calisthenics	0.0333	0.795	1.590	4.27
Golf (walking)	0.0360	0.540	1.080	4.62
Handball	0.0630	0.945	1.890	8.08
Hiking	0.0420	0.630	1.260	5.38
Paddleball	0.0690	1.035	2.070	8.85
Ping-Pong	0.0304	0.456	0.912	3.90
Running (cross country)	0.0740	1.110	2.220	9.49
Running (level track)				
4.5 mph (13:30 min./mi.)	0.0630	0.945	1.890	8.08
5.0 mph (12:00 min./mi.)	0.0667	0.999	1.999	8.55
5.5 mph (11:00 min./mi.)	0.0711	1.067	2.133	9.12
6.0 mph (10:00 min./mi.)	0.0790	1.185	2.370	10.13
7.0 mph (8:30 min./mi.)	0.0933	1.399	2.799	11.96
8.7 mph (6:54 min./mi.)	0.1031	1.547	3.094	13.22
10.0 mph (6:00 min./mi.)	0.1066	1.599	3.198	13.67
12.0 mph (5:00 min./mi.)	0.1311	1.967	3.933	16.81
Running (sprints)	0.1552	2.328	4.656	19.90
Squash	0.0691	1.037	2.074	8.86
Stationary running				
70-80 counts/min.	0.0780	1.170	2.340	10.00
140 counts/min.	0.1622	2.433	4.866	20.79

Adapted from C.F. Consolazio, R.E. Johnson, and L.J. Pecora, *Physiological measurements of metabolic functions in man* (New York: McGraw-Hill, 1963), pp. 331-32.

NOTE: The number of calories expended in any activity can be obtained by multiplying the number of calories per minute per pound by your weight and by the number of minutes the activity is performed.

*Based on an average caloric consumption of 1.2 Cal./min. for a 154-lb. man sitting at rest.

TABLE 6-9, CONTINUED

	Cal./lb.			
Activity	*1 Min.*	*15 Min.*	*30 Min.*	METS*
Swimming (pleasure)	0.0724	1.086	2.172	9.28
Breast stroke (20 yd./min.)	0.0319	0.479	0.958	4.09
Breast stroke (40 yd./min.)	0.0639	0.959	1.918	8.19
Back stroke (25 yd./min.)	0.0252	0.378	0.756	3.23
Back stroke (35 yd./min.)	0.0454	0.681	1.362	5.82
Side stroke (40 yd./min.)	0.0554	0.831	1.662	7.10
Crawl (45 yd./min.)	0.0580	0.870	1.740	7.44
Crawl (55 yd./min.)	0.0706	1.059	2.118	9.05
Tennis	0.0460	0.690	1.380	5.90
Volleyball	0.0233	0.350	0.699	2.99
Walking (level ground)				
2.27 mph (26:26 min./mi.)	0.0233	0.350	0.700	2.99
3.20 mph (18:45 min./mi.)	0.0313	0.470	0.940	4.01
3.50 mph (17:09 min./mi.)	0.0332	0.498	0.996	4.26
4.47 mph (13:25 min./mi.)	0.0524	0.786	1.572	6.72
4.60 mph (13:03 min./mi.)	0.0551	0.827	1.654	7.06
5.18 mph (11:35 min./mi.)	0.0627	0.941	1.882	8.04
5.80 mph (10:21 min./mi.)	0.0756	1.134	2.268	9.69

REFERENCES

1. American Heart Association. *The way to a man's heart.* New York: American Heart Association, 1972.
2. Brozek, J.; Grande, F.; Anderson, J.T.; and Keys, A. Densitometric analysis of body composition: Revision of some quantitative assumptions. *Annals of the New York Academy of Science* 110: 113-140, 1963.
3. Bucher, C.A.; Olsen, E.A.; and Willgoose, C.E. *The foundations of health.* New York: Appleton-Century-Crofts, 1967.
4. Burton, B.T. *The Heinz handbook of nutrition.* New York: McGraw-Hill, 1965.
5. Deutsch, R.M. *The family guide to better food and better health.* Des Moines: Meredith Corporation, 1971.
6. Fabry, P.; Hejl, Z.; Fodor, J.; Braun, T.; and Zvolankova, K. The frequency of meals: Its relation to overweight, hypercholesterolemia, and decreased glucose tolerance. *Lancet* 2: 614-615, 1964.
7. Hockey, R.V. *Physical fitness.* 2d ed. St. Louis: C.V. Mosby, 1973.
8. Johnson, P.B. *So you really want to lose weight?* Toledo: The University of Toledo, 1972. In Johnson, P.B.; Updike, W.F.; Schaefer, M.; and Stolberg, D.C. *Sport, exercise and you.* New York: Holt, Rinehart and Winston, 1975.
9. Johnson, P.B.; Updike, W.F.; Schaefer, M.; and Stolberg, D.C. *Sport, exercise and you.* New York: Holt, Rinehart and Winston, 1975.
10. Kimber, D.C.; Gray, C.E.; Stackpole, C.C.; and Leavell, L.C. *Anatomy and physiology.* New York: Macmillan, 1966.
11. Mayer, J. *Overweight: Causes, cost and control.* Englewood Cliffs: Prentice-Hall, 1968.
12. Neal, K.G. *Knowledge of health series.* Long Beach: ELOT Publishing, 1975.
13. Sheldon, W.; Stevens, S.S.; and Tucker, W.B. *The varieties of human physique.* Darien, Connecticut: Hafner, 1970.
14. Sloan, A.W. Estimation of body fat in young men. *Journal of Applied Physiology* 23: 311-315, 1967.
15. Sloan, A.W.; Burt, J.J.; and Blyth, C.S. Estimation of body fat in young women. *Journal of Applied Physiology* 17: 967-970, 1962.
16. White, P.L., and Selvy, N. *Let's talk about food.* Acton, Massachusetts: Publishing Sciences Group, 1974.
17. Zuti, W.B., and Golding, L.A. Comparing diet and exercise as weight reduction tools. *The Physician and Sports Medicine* 4: 49-53, January 1973.

KEY TERMS

Catecholamines (p. 105)
Homeostatic balance (p. 104)
Relaxation (p. 108)
Stress (p. 104)
Stressor (p. 104)
Sympathetic nervous system (p. 104)
Tension (p. 105)

BEHAVIORAL OBJECTIVES

Upon completion of this chapter the student
should be able to:

1. Define the key terms listed above.
2. Describe six body changes promoted by the
   sympathetic nervous system and the adrenal
   glands in response to a stressor.
3. Define *epinephrine* and *norepinephrine* and
   describe the effects of these substances.
4. Describe the tense individual.
5. List eight stress-related diseases and disorders.
6. Describe the role of exercise in the prevention
   of stress-related diseases.
7. Determine whether he or she is a tense
   individual.
8. Release tension through a relaxation
   technique.

CHAPTER SEVEN
STRESS

If the **homeostatic balance** (physiological equilibrium) of the body is disturbed, the individual experiences **stress**. Psychological as well as physiologic conditions can promote stress, but, whatever the cause, the body does not differentiate among the **stressors**. The reaction to emotional stress appears to be physiologically identical to the reaction induced by physical stress. It continues to exist in the body until homeostatic balance is restored.

Not everyone reacts the same to a stressful situation. Some individuals thrive on stress and actually rise to the occasion to function better mentally and physically; many top executives of major businesses fall in this category. In addition, certain individuals do not react emotionally to experiences that can be considered stressful. Their personalities appear to remain calm. However, others react strongly and become emotionally and physically disturbed. These people often have physical problems or disorders. The difference in the reactions of people to an emotional crisis is often due to the various ways in which different individuals perceive the stress. Some magnify the significance of an experience, while others are able to perceive that the experience may not be important.

Selye, a Canadian physician and endocrinologist, describes three stages the body goes through during stress (9). Initially, during the alarm reaction stage, the body reacts to stress. Changes in body chemistry take place to prepare the body for the stressful experience. This stage is followed by the resistance stage, in which the body attempts to adapt to the stress. If no adaptation takes place, the exhaustive stage follows, in which physical disorders, or possibly even death, are experienced.

BODY CHANGES

Sudden emotions of fear, anger, or excitement stimulate the **sympathetic nervous system** and the *adrenal glands* to instant action. The sympathetic nervous system produces the following changes in the body (1).

1. The heart rate and stroke volume are increased, which results in an increased cardiac output.
2. Blood vessels in the skin, kidneys, and most internal organs become constricted, which decreases the blood flow to these areas; blood vessels in the skeletal muscles become dilated, which increases the flow to them.
3. Systolic blood pressure and the volume of blood circulating per minute are increased.

4. Secretions and *peristalsis* of the digestive glands are decreased, and thus there is decreased digestion.
5. Liver glycogenolysis (breakdown of *glycogen* to glucose) is increased, which results in more blood glucose.
6. The breakdown of adipose-tissue triglyceride is increased.
7. The rate of ventilation is increased.
8. Muscle **tension** is increased.

There is also a rapid and marked rise in the amount of epinephrine (adrenaline) and norepinephrine secreted by the adrenal medulla. These two important secretions, known as **catecholamines**, help to increase and prolong the responses of the sympathetic nervous system. Epinephrine accelerates the rate and increases the strength of heart contraction, dilates coronary and skeletal muscle blood vessels, and constricts vessels in many other body organs; thus it raises blood pressure and redirects blood flow to areas with increased metabolic needs. Norepinephrine is almost exclusively a vasoconstrictor for the small blood vessels of muscle tissue (*peripheral circulation*) and plays a minor role in the increase in cardiac pumping.

Stress also initiates a series of reactions that stimulate the adrenal cortex to release the hormone cortisol. The functions of cortisol are as follows (11):

1. Stimulation of protein catabolism
2. Stimulation of the liver to convert amino acids to glucose
3. Inhibition of the oxidation of glucose by many body cells, but not by the brain

These body changes promoted by the sympathetic nervous system and the adrenal glands are ideally suited to cope with stressful experiences. When prehistoric humans were faced with emotionally exciting and physically demanding situations, they usually had to be prepared to fight for their lives or to run to save themselves. Either choice required action and placed demands upon the body. The sympathetic nervous system helped the cardiovascular and respiratory systems to supply oxygen and nutrients to the body cells and to remove waste products. The effects of cortisol enabled people to forego eating for a lengthy period of time, which they often had to do on occasions of danger. In addition, the amino acids liberated by the catabolism of body protein provided energy and a source for tissue repair if injury occurred. Today, these body changes continue to take place when people are confronted with stress. Recent evidence suggests that the secretion of almost every known hormone can be influenced by stress (11).

Emotional conflicts brought on by the many turmoils of our present society stimulate a person's glands, which prepare the body for a stressful experience. However, urban civilization makes it virtually impossible to relieve the tensions within the body, as people are not provided with motivation and opportunity for or social approval of the vigorous activities needed to neutralize hormone secretions. Modern society has made the fight-or-flight concept obsolete, but it has not changed the autonomic nervous system's response to stress. It is very possible that failure to understand this response contributes to the development of stress-induced diseases.

THE TENSE INDIVIDUAL

The muscles are arranged in pairs around each joint. As one member of the pair contracts, the other should relax. If the opposing muscle is under tension, it does not relax but resists movement, which results in wasted energy, further fatigue, and increased tension. The tense individual, expending vast amounts of energy without producing results other than fatigue, is therefore not a physically efficient person and is often very tired (6).

The habitually tense individual seeks to release tension in physical actions that are in no way related to the problem created by the tension — drumming the fingers on the table aimlessly or forcibly to express irritation; continually moving in the chair in attempts to find a comfortable position; twisting a lock of hair, scratching the scalp, or pulling at an ear; gripping a pencil until the fingers become numb; twisting a handkerchief or clasping the hands in a deathlike grip; twitching the face or assuming expressions of intense concentration, grinding the teeth, and shrugging the shoulders. Sitting "motionless," the tense individual twists a ring about the finger, crosses and uncrosses the legs, and wraps the feet around each other. Movement and posture appear stiff. Such a person complains of being tired, worries, and easily becomes angry or frustrated if faced with a problem for which there is no immediate solution (6).

STRESS-RELATED DISEASES AND DISORDERS

Emotional stress without meaningful physical movement has very detrimental effects on the body. It increases the levels of fatty acids in the blood stream, and hence it is related to atherosclerotic problems (9). Prolonged tension, if frequently repeated, can lead to insomnia, colitis, and hypertension. Digestion is inhibited, and acid enters the stomach, which leads to ulcers. Constipation, high serum cholesterol, and shortened time of blood coagulation are also consequences of emotional stress without physical movement. The muscle tightness that usually accompanies unpleasant emotions can create back, neck, chest, and stomach pains. Other symptoms of stress include headache, fuzzy vision, loss of appetite, and depression. Indeed, Selye's theory of stress postulates that almost any disease can be caused by emotional tension.

ROLE OF PHYSICAL EXERCISE

People are designed to be physically active, and many experts believe that movement can help prevent stress-related diseases and problems. Some studies indicate that fat is cleared more rapidly from the blood after exercise and that a physical training program increases this effect; this serves to prevent atherosclerosis (12).

Michael (7) found that moderate exercise actually provides a mild type of stress for the adrenal glands, which helps to condition and fortify them so that they can manage severe stresses more effectively. The increased adrenal activity that results from repeated exercise seems to cause the formation of greater reserves of steroids, which are suitable for counteracting stress.

Other studies have indicated that repeated physical exercise decreases catecholamine uptake by the trained heart (8). The heart responds to catecholamines with an increased pulse rate and an augmented coronary blood flow. However, the trained heart is more efficient in this response and more sensitive to the increased oxygen need, and thus it wastes less myocardial oxygen.

Studies involving mentally ill patients have verified that sports and moderate physical activity have value in the release of tension. DeVries (5) concluded that rhythmic exercise, such as walking, jogging, cycling, and bench-stepping, with durations of 5 to 30 minutes and intensities of 30% to 60% of maximum heart rate promotes significant relaxation for the tense individual. Also, through concentration on the game and on the opponent, tennis players, handball players, and participants in similar activities find a mental diversion that provides their worried minds with a new set of problems to solve; solutions to these problems, however, can be found in a short space of time. Habitual worry or anxiety is temporarily forgotten, and physical tensions arising from these concerns are released (4).

Selye (9) classifies exercise as a potent stressor. In the first stage, the body responds to the demands of exercise. Through training and progressive amounts of reasonable exercise, an efficient response results, and the exhaustion phase of stress is deterred. Selye suggests that an individual who exercises regularly should be better prepared to resist other stressors and that stressful situations are not as dangerous to a physically conditioned individual as to a sedentary individual.

Socially acceptable outlets for natural aggressive drives provide important physical and emotional benefits. Anger, hate, and frustration, often excluded from open expression by society, can be transformed into running, swimming, tennis, golf, or many other forms of physical activity, and this results in a healthier and happier life.

TECHNIQUES FOR RELAXATION

Relaxation is a conscious release of muscular tension. It is a skill that is based on an awareness of the presence of tension, and it is one that is not easily performed by many individuals. These individuals must learn to relax in much the same way that they would learn any other motor skill (10).

Various relaxation techniques have been reported to be successful in the release of tension. Benson (3) proposed the following technique:

1. Sit quietly in a comfortable position and close the eyes.
2. Beginning at the feet and progressing to the head, relax all the muscles.
3. Breathe through the nose. Each time you breathe out, silently say the word *one.* Breathe easily and naturally.
4. Continue for 10 to 20 minutes. You may occasionally check the time, but do not use an alarm. When you finish, sit quietly for several minutes.
5. Maintain a positive attitude and permit relaxation to occur at its own pace. When distracting thoughts occur, try to ignore them by not dwelling upon them, and continue to repeat the word *one.*

Arnheim et al. (2) reported a more involved relaxation technique.

1. Assume a supine position on a firm mat with each body curve (i.e., the neck, elbows, lower back, and knees) comfortably supported by a pillow or a towel. The arms should be spread so that they do not contact the clothing or the body. Take five deep breaths; inhale and exhale slowly.
2. Curl the toes down and point the feet downward. Do not bite down hard with the teeth or hold the breath. Relax. Try to relax all other parts as you tense one area of the body.

3. Curl the toes and the feet back toward the head. Breathe easily and relax.

4. Press down against the floor with the heels and attempt to curl the legs backward. Relax.

5. Straighten the legs to full extension. Let go and breathe easily.

6. Draw the thighs up to a bent position and raise the heels off the floor about 3 in. Tension should be felt in the bend of the hip. Return slowly to the starting position and relax.

7. Forcibly rotate the thighs outward. Feel the tension in the outer hip region. Relax.

8. Rotate the thighs inward. Feel the tension deep in the inner thighs. Relax slowly and let the thighs again rotate outward.

9. Squeeze the buttocks together tightly and tilt the hips backward. Tension should be felt in the buttocks and also in the lower back. Relax.

10. Tighten the abdominal muscles and flatten the lower back. Tension should be felt in both areas. Relax.

11. Inhale and exhale slowly and deeply three times. Return to normal quiet breathing.

12. Press the head back and lift the upper back off the floor. The tension should be felt in the back of the neck and the upper back. Relax.

13. Squeeze the shoulder blades together. Tension should be felt in the back of the shoulders. Relax.

14. Leaving the arms in their resting position, lift and roll the shoulders inward so that tension is felt in the front of the chest. Relax.

15. Spread and clinch the fingers of both hands three times. Relax.

16. Make tight fists with both hands and slowly curl the wrists back, forward, and to both sides. Allow the fingers and thumbs to open gradually and relax.

17. Make tight fists with both hands and slowly flex the forearm against the upper arm. At the same time, lift the arm at the shoulder. Slowly uncurl the arms and return them to their original resting position. Relax.

18. Make tight fists with both hands, stiffen the arms, and press hard against the floor. Hold the pressure for 30 seconds. Slowly relax.

19. Shrug the right shoulder. Bend the head sideward and touch the ear to the elevated shoulder. Slowly relax.

20. Repeat step 19 with the left shoulder.

21. Bend the head forward and touch the chin to the chest. Slowly relax.

22. Lift the eyebrows upward and wrinkle the forehead. Let the face go blank.
23. Close the eyelids tightly and wrinkle the nose. Relax the face slowly.
24. Open the mouth widely, as if to yawn. Slowly relax.
25. Bite down hard, and then show the teeth in a forced smile. Slowly relax.
26. Pucker the lips in a whistle position. Slowly relax.
27. Push the tongue hard against the roof of the mouth. Relax. Perform this three times.
28. Move slowly and take any position desired. Relax and rest.

With practice, either of the above techniques can be successful in the promotion of relaxation. Individuals who have difficulty in the attainment of a relaxed state should use a technique that provides the best success for them.

REFERENCES

1. Anthony, C.P., and Kolthoff, N.J. *Anatomy and physiology.* 9th ed. St. Louis: C.V. Mosby, 1975.
2. Arnheim, D.D.; Auxter, D.; and Crowe, W.C. *Principles and methods of adapted physical education.* St. Louis: C.V. Mosby, 1969.
3. Benson, H. *The relaxation response.* New York: William Morrow and Company, 1975.
4. Byrd, O. Studies on the psychological values of lifetime sports. *Journal of Health, Physical Education, Recreation* 38: 35-36, November-December 1967.
5. deVries, H.A. Physical education, adult fitness programs: Does physical activity promote relaxation? *Journal of Physical Education and Recreation* 46: 53-54, 1975.
6. Methany, E. *Body dynamics.* New York: McGraw-Hill, 1952.
7. Michael, E.D. Stress adaptation through exercise. *Research Quarterly* 28: 50-54, 1957.
8. President's Council on Physical Fitness and Sports. Effects of chronic exercise on cardiovascular function. *Physical Fitness Research Digest.* Edited by H.H. Clarke. Series 2, No. 3, July 1972.
9. Selye, H. *The stress of life.* New York: McGraw-Hill, 1956.
10. Scott, M.A. *Analysis of human motion.* 2nd ed. New York: Appleton-Century-Crofts, 1963.
11. Vander, A.J., Sherman, J.H.; and Luciano, D.S. *Human physiology — the mechanism of body function.* 2d ed. New York: McGraw-Hill, 1975.
12. Watt, J. Exercise and heart disease — related fields of research. In *Exercise and Fitness.* Edited by S.C. Staley, T.K. Cureton, L.J. Huelster, and A.J. Barry. Chicago: Athletic Institute, 1960.

KEY TERMS

Accelerator nerve (p. 113)
Aorta (p. 112)
Atria (p. 112)
Atrioventricular (A-V) node (p. 114)
Atrioventricular (A-V) valve (p. 112)
Bundle of His (p. 114)
Chordae tendineae (p. 112)
Diastasis (p. 115)
Diastole (p. 115)
Interventricular septum (p. 114)
Murmurs (p. 116)
Myocardium (p. 112)
Pulmonary artery (p. 112)
Pulmonary veins (p. 112)
Purkinje fibers (p. 114)
Semilunar valves (p. 112)
Sino-auricular (S-A) node (p. 114)
Systole (p. 115)
Vagus nerve (p. 113)
Venae cavae (p. 112)
Ventricles (p. 112)

BEHAVIORAL OBJECTIVES

Upon completion of this chapter, the student should be able to:

1. Define or identify the key terms.
2. Make a schematic diagram of the heart and label the following structures:
   a. Right and left atria
   b. Right and left ventricles
   c. Pacemaker, A-V node
   d. Interventricular septum
   e. Myocardium
   f. Pulmonary artery, pulmonary veins
   g. Aorta
   h. Superior and inferior venae cavae
   i. Mitral and tricuspid valves
   j. Pulmonic and aortic valves
   k. Papillary muscles and chordae tendineae
3. Trace blood flow from right atrium to aorta; list in order the structures passed.
4. Identify basic events of the cardiac cycle and causes of the first and second heart sounds.
5. List four acute and four long-term effects of exercise on the cardiovascular system.
6. List normal values for resting heart rate, systolic blood pressure, diastolic blood pressure, stroke volume, and cardiac output.
7. List maximal normal values for heart rate and systolic blood pressure.

CHAPTER EIGHT
CIRCULATION

HEART
BLOOD

The ability of one's heart and vascular system to deliver blood with its oxygen to active muscle tissue appears, at present, to be the most important limitation of exercise. Although there is a high rate of energy turnover during cardiac work, the mechanical efficiency of the heart per beat is very low. Nevertheless, the amount of work accomplished by this small organ without cessation or breakdown is astonishing. It has been calculated that the work performed by a normal heart during one's lifetime is the equivalent of lifting a 30-ton weight to a height of 30,000 ft. (2).

BASIC STRUCTURE

As can be seen in Figure 8-1, the heart is a hollow organ composed of four chambers. The upper chambers are identified as the left and right **atria**, and the lower chambers are the **ventricles. Atrioventricular (A-V) valves** connect the atria with the ventricles. Attached to the cusps of these valves are tendinous cords (**chordae tendineae**), which are in turn attached to small muscles located on the inner walls of the ventricles. These structures prevent inversion of the A-V valves under the high pressures created by the pumping action of the heart. The **semilunar valves** are located at the roots of the **aorta** and the **pulmonary artery**. These valves prevent a backflow of blood during the relaxation phase of the cardiac cycle.

Cardiac Vessels

The superior and inferior **venae cavae** return blood from the upper and lower extremities, respectively, to the right atrium. The pulmonary artery delivers blood from the right ventricle to the lungs, and **pulmonary veins** complete the circuit between the lungs and the left atrium. From the left ventricle, the aorta, the largest artery in the body, transports the blood through its branches to all parts of the body. It is important to understand that these vessels (except the aorta) deliver blood to the chambers of the heart for pumping purposes only; none of this blood is actually used by the **myocardium** (heart muscle) as a source of oxygen. Oxygen and other nutrients necessary for myocardial metabolism must come by way of the coronary arteries and their branches, which encircle and perfuse the myocardium. (See Figure 8-2.)

1. Superior vena cava
2. Inferior vena cava
3. Sino-auricular node (pacemaker)
4. Right atrium
5. Atrio-ventricular node
6. Tricuspid valve
7. Chordae tendineae
8. Papillary muscle
9. Right ventricle
10. Pulmonic valve
11. Pulmonary artery
12. Pulmonary veins
13. Left atrium
14. Mitral valve
15. Left ventricle
16. Aortic valve
17. Aorta
18. Interventricular septum
19. Ventricular myocardium

Figure 8-1. The heart.

Cardiac Innervation

The heart itself is capable of contraction independent of any extrinsic nerve supply. However, two external cardiac nerves are important. The **accelerator nerve**, which belongs to the sympathetic division of the autonomic nervous system, provides stimuli that increase heart rate. The **vagus nerve** presents stimuli from the para-

1. Right CA
2. Left main CA
3. Left anterior descending CA
4. Left circumflex CA

Figure 8-2. Coronary arteries (CA).

sympathetic division of the autonomic nervous system and serves to reduce heart rate.

The pacing (rhythm) of the heart is normally determined by the activity of the **sino-auricular node** (also called the **S-A node,** *sinus node*, or *pacemaker*), located in the right atrium near the superior vena cava. This mass of nervous tissue sends out an electrical stimulus, which is conducted by the muscle cells of the atria, and which results in atrial contraction. As the contraction wave reaches the **atrioventricular (A-V) node**, in the base of the right atrium near the **interventricular septum**, it is transmitted through the ventricular myocardium over a well-defined nerve network composed of the **Purkinje fibers** and the **Bundle of His.** Besides these major rhythm-regulating nodes, there are other nodes, located throughout the myocardium, that can produce contraction in the event of a failure of the S-A or

A-V nodes. Occasionally, one or more of these nodes becomes irritable and fires at random; this produces extra contractions, which are sometimes felt as extra beats or "skipped" beats. These are usually harmless but sometimes disturbing to the owner. In such cases, it is wise to consult a physician for accurate diagnosis. Equally important in such cases is the early establishment of an electrocardiographic base line, which can be helpful in the diagnosis of the relative severity or innocence of similar occurrences that might manifest themselves later. The reasons for these occasional innocent "short circuits" are not well understood, but the increased nodal irritability that produces them is thought to be associated with cigarette smoking, use of drinks that contain caffeine, and lack of rest.

CARDIAC CYCLE

In attempting to understand the relation among the events of the cardiac cycle, one should be aware that the atria work as a unit, as do the ventricles; therefore, an occurrence on one side of the heart almost simultaneously takes place on the other side. It should also be understood that the right and left sides of the heart serve somewhat different functions. The right side receives deoxygenated blood (blood with a relatively high content of carbon dioxide and a somewhat reduced oxygen content) from the body, pumps it to the lungs to be oxygenated, and returns it to the left atrium. The left side receives this freshly oxygenated blood from the lungs via the pulmonary veins and pumps it to all parts of the body under enough pressure to ensure its return to the right atrium. Obviously, a much higher pressure must be generated by the left side of the heart — approximately five times as high as that developed by the right side — and, accordingly, the wall of the left side is much thicker and stronger.

The mechanical events that promote blood flow through the heart and the cardiovascular system can be classified in three categories, which characterize the three phases of the cardiac cycle. They are: (1) **systole**, or contraction, (2) **diastole**, or relaxation, and (3) **diastasis**, or rest. These terms designate the state of the myocardial fibers at different times in the cycle. Each phase first occurs in the atria and then spreads to the ventricles. Although ventricular systole follows atrial systole very closely, the two do not occur simultaneously. The contracting, relaxing, and resting of the heart muscle, together with effective action of the valves, create pressure differentials between the chambers, which facilitate blood flow in the proper direction.

In describing the events of the cardiac cycle, one might begin at any point so long as the proper sequence is followed, e.g., diastole, diastasis, systole. Increases in heart rate can alter the relative amount of time allowed for a particular phase or can even eliminate diastasis completely; however, the normal sequence of events is unaffected.

Beginning with atrial diastasis, a sketchy account of the most important events of the cardiac cycle reads as follows: During atrial diastasis, the fibers encircling the atria are at rest, the A-V valves are open, and blood flows freely from the atria to the ventricles. At the outset of atrial systole, the stimulus from the pacemaker initiates contraction of the atrial fibers (atrial systole), which forces any blood that has collected in the atria into the ventricles. This ejection phase is followed by atrial diastole, at which time the atria are refilled. Even while the atria are contracting, the signal of the pacemaker is picked up by the A-V node and is distributed to the ventricular myocardium, which initiates ventricular systole. At the outset of this phase, the A-V valves, which were floated nearly closed during late diastole, are slammed tightly shut; since the semilunar valves are also closed, ventricular blood is trapped. The sound thus produced is fairly low-pitched and is caused in part by vibrations set up in the walls of the heart and the blood vessels by the closure of the valves. It is known as the *first heart sound*. The pressure in the ventricles continues to build under increasing myocardial tension until it is greater than the pressure in the adjacent ventricular artery. At this time, the semilunar valves are forced open and the ventricles eject their blood. Immediately after ventricular systole, the fibers begin to relax, which marks the beginning of ventricular diastole. Pressure in the ventricle becomes lower than that in the aorta and the pulmonary artery, and the semilunar valves slam shut. The sound thus created is the *second heart sound*; it is higher pitched and more crisp than the first. If a valve is structurally or functionally abnormal, additional sounds (**murmurs**) usually accompany the normal heart sounds. (See page 13.)

VASCULAR SYSTEM

To assist the heart in the delivery of blood throughout the body, three types of vessels are employed — arteries, veins, and capillaries. Functionally, the arteries carry blood away from the heart; the veins return the blood to the heart; the capillaries are the connecting links between the arterial and venous trees, which allow respiratory gases

TABLE 8-1
CHARACTERISTICS OF ARTERIES, VEINS, AND CAPILLARIES

Vessel	Size	Characteristics
Arteries	30 μ-2.5 cm	Walls thicker than those of corresponding veins
		Muscle tissue thicker than that in corresponding veins
		No apparent diffusion through walls
Veins	20 μ-3.0 cm	Walls thinner than those of corresponding arteries
		Muscle tissue thinner than that in corresponding arteries
		Valves present in larger veins
		No apparent diffusion through walls
Capillaries	1 μ-8 μ	Walls one cell thick, freely permit diffusion

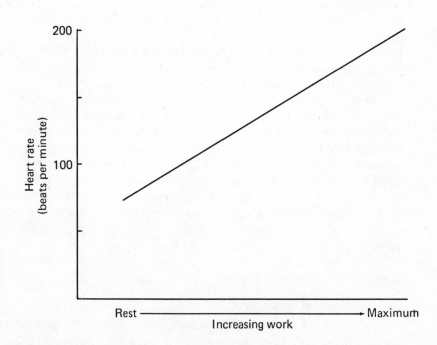

Figure 8-3. Heart rate response to increasing work loads.

and nutrients to be exchanged freely between the cells and the circulating blood. The duties of these vessels dictate that they be structurally different. Some of these differences are shown in Table 8-1.

CARDIOVASCULAR RESPONSES TO EXERCISE

Any discussion of cardiovascular responses to exercise must be qualified in terms of acute effects or long-term effects, because these types of responses are quite different. Furthermore, the kind of exercise employed is an important consideration. In this chapter, any reference to exercise or training should be taken to mean dynamic exercise (e.g., running or swimming) strenuous enough to elevate the heart rate to a sustained 140 to 150 beats per minute for at least 5 to 10 minutes.

To study circulatory responses to exercise, certain circulatory parameters, such as heart rate, blood pressure, stroke volume, and cardiac output, are measured when the subject is at rest, and again during submaximal and maximal exercise; comparisons are then made. It is generally accepted that the resting untrained heart averages 70 to 80 beats per minute; however, these values may range from 50 to 90 beats per minutes and still not indicate a pathologic condition. The typical heart rate of females is between 5 and 8 beats per minute higher than the rate typical for males. This may be because in females the heart is somewhat smaller in relation to body size, and so is the stroke output per beat. If the average volume ejected per stroke (70 to 80 ml) is multiplied by the average heart rate (70 to 80 beats per minute), the resulting output of the heart per minute (cardiac output) is approximately 4 to 6 ℓ of blood. The pressure generated by this outflow of blood against the artery walls is known as arterial blood pressure. Arterial pressure is pulsatile, as is demonstrated by its elevation when the heart contracts and its fall when the heart relaxes. The peak pressure measured during contraction (systolic pressure) averages about 120 ± 20 mm Hg in normal subjects. The pressure measured during relaxation of the ventricle (diastolic pressure) is lower; it averages about 80 ± 10 mm Hg.

Acute Effects of Exercise

As an individual begins to exercise, the heart rate increases linearly in proportion to the severity of the work. If the work is not maximal, the heart rate reaches a plateau after about 3 to 5 minutes and continues at that level for several minutes, again in proportion to the work load. This elevated heart rate is the result of an increased oxygen demand at the cellular level by the exercising muscles. The ultimate goal of the cardiovascular system is to increase cardiac output and thereby increase the delivery of blood to the areas that need it so that a balance between oxygen demanded and oxygen supplied can be achieved. This is accomplished by one or all of the following compensatory adjustments:

1. Increase in the heart rate
2. Increase in the stroke volume
3. Increase in the perfusion of the exercising tissue by means of flow through previously unopened capillaries
4. Increase in the amount of oxygen extracted from the blood by the working cells

Most people can elevate the effective heart rate to between two and three times the resting rate. In a majority of cases, the heart rate range (maximum rate minus resting rate) amounts to about 100 beats per minute, since 170 or 180 beats per minute is thought by many to be the greatest effective heart rate even though 200 and 210 beats per minute are not uncommon in individuals below age 20 (1).

The heart becomes a stronger pump due to the liberation of certain substances called *catecholamines*, which enable it to clear its ventricles more completely. As a result, stroke volume can be increased from 70 ml (when the individual is at rest) to almost double that amount (when the individual engages in heavy exercise).

In addition to these two adjustments, the capillary beds in the working muscles can open more completely, to allow approximately three times more blood to enter; also, *oxygen extraction* from a given volume of blood can be increased. Considering the combined effects of these adjustments, one can expect at least a 12-fold increase in the amount of blood delivered to the exercising tissue, in comparison with what is supplied during resting conditions.

During exercise, the systolic pressure in normal subjects increases linearly with the work load to a maximum value of about 240 mm Hg. The normal diastolic-pressure response to physical effort is less predictable; it might increase or decrease slightly or remain unchanged. In trained subjects, a slight decrease is usually observed as peripheral vascular resistance drops. In any case, an increase of more than 15 mm Hg over the resting diastolic pressure is considered a hypertensive response.

It has been shown that arm work elicits higher blood pressures, ventilatory volumes, and heart rates than does work by the legs for an equivalent work load (3). The significance of this finding applied to everyday life is that, since cardiovascular stress is greater during arm work, middle-aged, untrained individuals should be extremely cautious about sporadic heavy work with the arms (e.g., shoveling snow or dirt, loading heavy items, or rowing). Furthermore, isometric work (straining against heavy resistance) should be discouraged, particularly in older people, because of the extremely high blood pressures this type of activity produces.

Long-Term Effects of Exercise

If the body is exposed to regular bouts of exercise of sufficient intensity and duration, physiologic adaptation occurs, which improves one's ability to tolerate similar amounts of work with less difficulty. Well-documented cardiovascular responses to long-term endurance training are as follows:

1. Reduced resting heart rate
2. Reduced exercise heart rate for all submaximal work
3. Increased stroke volume at rest, during submaximal work, and during maximal work   *heart rate x volume*
4. Increased cardiac output during maximal work

Other training-induced changes that have been reported, but which remain controversial, include reductions in the levels of blood lipids, such as serum triglycerides and serum cholesterol, increases in the number of capillaries per unit of tissue, and improvements in *collateral circulation* in the myocardium. Tables 4-1 and 4-2 in Chapter 4 summarize these and other training-induced changes.

REFERENCES

1. Astrand, P.O., and Rodahl, K. *Textbook of work physiology.* 2d ed. New York: McGraw-Hill, 1977.
2. Burton, A.C. *Physiology and biophysics of the circulation.* Chicago: Year Book Medical Publishers, 1965.
3. Clausen, J.P.; Trap-Jensen, J.; and Lassen, N.A. The effects of training in the heart rate during arm and leg exercise. *Scandinavian Journal of Clinical and Laboratory Investigation* 26: 295-301, 1970.
4. Franklin, M.; Krauthamer, M.; Tai, A.R.; and Pinchot, A. *The heart doctors' heart book.* New York: Bantam Books, 1976.
5. Guyton, A.C. *Textbook of medical physiology.* 5th ed. Philadelphia: W.B. Saunders, 1977.
6. Rushmer, R.F. *Cardiovascular dynamics.* Philadelphia: W.B. Saunders, 1970.

KEY TERMS
Aerobic capacity (p. 124)
Aerobic metabolism (p. 125)
Anaerobic metabolism (p. 125)
Maximum oxygen uptake (p. 124)
Oxygen debt (p. 125)
Pulmonary ventilation (p. 122)
Steady state (p. 125)

BEHAVIORAL OBJECTIVES
Upon completion of this chapter the student
should be able to:
1. Define the key terms listed above.
2. Describe orally or in writing the mechanism of
   oxygen delivery to the cells.
3. Identify the adjustments the respiratory
   system makes during exercise.
4. Describe the changes in respiratory function
   that result from long-term endurance training.

CHAPTER NINE
RESPIRATION

It is unrealistic to discuss the role of the circulatory system in exercise and training without a treatment of the contributions of the respiratory system as well. In fact, increasing one's ability to deliver blood to working tissue is quite futile without a concomitant improvement in the respiratory system. Fortunately, the two systems are related, so that activities that develop either one also stimulate improvement in the other. Therefore, many writers combine the systems and speak of the *circulorespiratory (CR) system.*

BASIC COMPONENTS OF THE RESPIRATORY SYSTEM

The basic components of the respiratory system are as follows:
1. Entryways (mouth and nose)
2. Trachea (windpipe)
3. Primary bronchi
4. Lungs (composed of many branches and subdivisions of *bronchioles* through about 23 generations, and finally terminating in a *respiratory bronchiole* with its alveolar sacs)

Figure 9-1 shows these structures along with several important surrounding structures that enclose the lung in the thoracic cavity and that assist breathing.

MECHANICS OF BREATHING

Breathing, also called **pulmonary ventilation**, consists of inhaling air (21% oxygen and 0.04% carbon dioxide) and exhaling lung air (14.2% oxygen and 5.5% carbon dioxide). At rest, inspiration is actively assisted by muscular contraction, while expiration is passive. The mechanics of the system require that inspiration occur when the *intercostal muscles* and the *diaphragm* contract. This causes the size of the thoracic cavity to increase, and therefore the lungs also expand, since they are attached to the wall by means of the pleura. The increase in volume results in a decrease in intrathoracic pressure, and if the passages to the lungs are unobstructed, air flows in to equalize the pressure.

The lungs are elastic and are stretched by the contraction of the respiratory musculature. Consequently, the relaxation of the muscles of respiration results in diminished thoracic size and elastic recoil of the lung tissue, which increases intrathoracic pressure and drives air out of the lungs. During exercise, however, when the lungs need to be emptied more rapidly or more completely than during rest, additional muscles are brought into play.

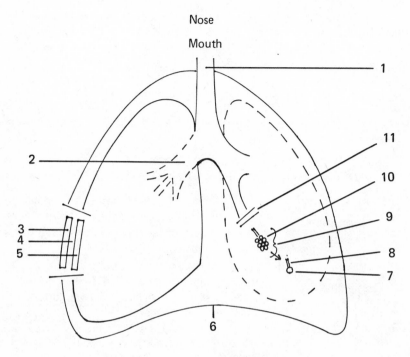

Nose

Mouth

1. Trachea
2. Bronchus
3. Parietal pleura
4. Pleural cavity
5. Visceral pleura
6. Diaphragm

7. Alveolus
8. Respiratory bronchiole
9. Alveolar sacs
10. Terminal bronchiole
11. Approximately 23 generations of branching omitted

Figure 9-1. The lung.

LUNG VOLUMES

A normal adult lung holds maximally about 6,200 to 7,400 ml of air. (The actual figure depends on certain body dimensions of the subject.) However, about 1,200 ml of that air (*residual air*) is never expelled from the lungs. This means that the maximum amount of air that can be expired after a maximum inspiration (*vital capacity*) is about 4,500 to 6,000 ml for men and 3,000 to 4,500 ml for women. During normal breathing, while the subject is at rest, only a small portion (about 500 ml) is inspired and expired (exchanged) during one respiratory cycle (inspiration plus expiration). This amount is referred to as *tidal air*.

If the normal respiratory frequency is assumed to be between 8 and 18 respirations per minute and the average tidal volume to be 500 ml, it is quite easy to calculate the *minute ventilatory volume* by the formula

$$\dot{V}_E = V_T \times f$$

where $\dot{V}_E$ = pulmonary ventilation, V_T = tidal volume, and f = respiratory frequency.

OXYGEN AND CARBON DIOXIDE TRANSPORT

The primary function of the CR system is the delivery of oxygen to cells in the quantity demanded by metabolic activity at a particular site. Equally important is the removal of carbon dioxide and other by-products of metabolism. The hemoglobin in circulating blood plays the major role in this oxygen/carbon dioxide transport function. As a result of differences in pressure of oxygen and carbon dioxide in the lungs and pulmonary capillaries and at the cellular level, diffusion gradients are established. These gradients, whose effects are enhanced by the affinity of hemoglobin for the two gases, facilitate its loading with oxygen and unloading of carbon dioxide in the capillaries of the lung and its unloading of oxygen and loading with carbon dioxide at the cellular level.

Under normal conditions of health and at normal atmospheric pressure, blood is about 98% saturated with oxygen when it leaves the lung. In a resting subject, about 30% of this oxygen is removed at the cellular level, but, during heavy exercise, this value can be increased almost three times. The amount of oxygen extracted from circulating blood in 1 minute is termed *oxygen uptake*. If measured during maximal exercise, this quantity is **maximum oxygen uptake**, which is believed by exercise physiologists to be the best single indicator of physical fitness, because it represents the ability of the body to mobilize all its systems during physical stress.

OXYGEN REQUIREMENT

Oxygen consumption ($\dot{V}O_2$) in an individual at rest is about 0.25 ℓ/min., or about 3.5 ml/kg/min. (The latter expression takes body weight into account.) During heavy exercise, this value can be increased 12 to 16 times depending on the relative state of CR fitness. The maximum $\dot{V}O_2$ that one can attain (**aerobic capacity**) measures the effectiveness of the heart, lungs, and vascular system in the delivery of oxygen during heavy work — the higher the $\dot{V}O_2$ max, the more effective the system.

One of the highest maximum oxygen uptakes on record is 6.2 ℓ/min. or 88 ml/kg/min., which was measured in a Scandinavian cross-country skier. Values reported in liters per minute, however, are useless for interpersonal comparisons, because these comparisons must take into account differences in body size. To adjust for body size, therefore, $\dot{V}O_2$ in liters per minute is divided by body weight in kilograms. The result is then reported in milliliters per kilogram per minute and can be used to compare individuals. By these data, subjects can be classified into poor, fair, and excellent, or into some similar categories based on $\dot{V}O_2$ max. (See Appendix, p. 149.)

OXYGEN DEBT

For cellular metabolism to continue for very long, adequate oxygen must be supplied (**aerobic metabolism**). This is not always possible, however. Two examples in which the supply is inadequate occur (1) at the beginning of heavy work, when the oxygen demand is greater than the response capability of the transport system, and (2) during prolonged heavy work at a very high intensity, when the oxygen demand is greater than the transport capacity of the cardiovascular system. In either case, the body is capable of working for short periods because of a wonderful and necessary process called **anaerobic metabolism**. When the body operates anaerobically, an **oxygen debt** is created, which must be repaid at a later time. Small oxygen debts are formed each time one deviates appreciably from the resting state, but these are rapidly repaid when the exercise ceases, because little or no *lactic acid* (a by-product of anaerobic metabolism) accumulates.

During work that requires less than 50% of one's aerobic capacity, the oxygen transport system is usually able to supply adequate amounts of oxygen to working tissue. When this happens, heart rate, ventilation, and $\dot{V}O_2$ can be maintained at a constant level for indefinite periods of time. This constitutes a balance between supply and demand and is termed **steady state.**

If, however, one engages in work that demands more than 50% of the aerobic capacity, the oxygen transport system is unable to supply as much as is demanded, and an oxygen debt is created. Anaerobic pathways of energy production are called into play, so that the invidual can continue working. This allows continued short-term performance, but working time is signifcantly reduced as lactic acid rapidly builds up. When the oxygen debt reaches about 15 ℓ, work must cease to allow for repayment and removal of some of the metabolic wastes that accumulated during the anaerobic work.

RECOVERY AFTER EXERCISE

One is fully recovered after exercise only when blood pressure, heart rate, ventilation, and $\dot{V}O_2$ have returned to preexercise levels. The amount of time required for recovery is a function of the intensity and the duration of the exercise and the relative state of training of the individual. One recovers faster if the oxygen debt incurred during the exercise is a moderate one, in which the *lactacid* component is very small.

EFFECTS OF EXERCISE ON THE RESPIRATORY SYSTEM

The immediate effects of exercise on the respiratory system demonstrate intensification of the ventilatory process. They are manifested in (1) an increase in respiratory frequency, (2) an increase in tidal volume, (3) an increase in the extent of the ventilated areas of the lung, and (4) an increase in the perfusion of the lung with blood. The magnitude of any increase is almost linearly related to the intensity of the exercise.

After several weeks of physical endurance training at an appropriate level, the respiratory function of an individual is improved in the following respects:

1. The maximum amount of air one can move per unit of time (*maximum voluntary ventilation*) is greater, owing to increases in both the strength and the endurance of the respiratory musculature.
2. Maximum oxygen uptake is increased.
3. Ventilation for identical submaximal work loads is decreased.
4. The pulmonary diffusing capacity during maximal work is increased.

RESPIRATORY PHENOMENA

Several interesting respiratory phenomena appear from time to time in some individuals and are therefore worthy of mention in a manual of this kind.

Second Wind

During the early minutes of vigorous work, uncomfortably difficult breathing (dyspnea) may occur. In some individuals, accompanying characteristics such as dizziness, heavy legs, chest pain, and general physical discomfort are also reported. However, after a few minutes of continuous work at the same intensity, these symptoms seem to disappear, the distress subsides, and one experiences a "second wind." This phenomenon is more common in untrained persons than in well-trained athletes, in whom it is rarely observed. The generally accepted explanation for second wind is that respiratory adaptation to work takes effect only after a time lag due to inadequate chemical regulation of respiration, so that metabolites accumulate in respiratory and working muscles during this lag.

Side Stitch

A side stitch often develops in untrained persons during running activities. This is manifested in excruciating pain in the area of the lower rib cage and is usually confined to the right side of the body. Several explanations have been offered, none of which are completely satisfactory. It is probable that all of the following factors contribute to the discomfort:

1. Accumulation of metabolic wastes (lactic acid) in the diaphragm
2. Severe shaking of the abdominal contents, which causes pain in the supporting structures
3. Formation of gas in the ascending colon
4. Reduced blood flow to the affected area due to the rerouting of blood to other areas

As is the case with second wind, side stitch rarely occurs in trained individuals. Relief appears to be hastened by the application of pressure on the affected side while the exercise is continued. If the pain becomes too severe, the only alternative is to terminate the work.

VENTILATION DURING RUNNING

Runners are often concerned about the efficiency of their methods of ventilating the lungs during exercise. They wonder whether they should breathe faster as the demands of exercise increase or whether they should breathe deeper. While the answer is not clear for all levels of exercise, some insight into the problem might be gained from the following example.

Assume that a runner at rest is breathing at a rate (f) of 10 times per minute and at a depth (V_T) of 0.5 ℓ per breath. From the ventilation equation found on page 124, it can be seen that the pulmonary ventilation ($\dot{V}_E$) is 5.0 ℓ/min.

$$\dot{V}_E = V_T \times f$$
$$= 0.5 \text{ ℓ/breath} \times 10 \text{ breaths/min.}$$
$$= 5.0 \text{ ℓ/min.}$$

Suppose that, during exercise, the runner's ventilatory demand increases to 20 ℓ/min. The question is whether the demand should be satisfied by an increase in V_T or in f, or both. At this low level, the answer clearly favors an increase in the depth (V_T) if the runner's desire is to remain efficient. The reason concerns repeated movement of dead space air (DSA) and can be explained as follows:

Although pulmonary ventilation describes the air flow to and from the lungs, alveolar ventilation ($\dot{V}_A$) represents the portion of pulmonary ventilation that actually reaches the alveolar level to participate in the oxygen/carbon dioxide exchange with pulmonary capillary blood. DSA is the volume of air that is contained in the respiratory passageways. Since it amounts roughly to 1 ml/lb. of body weight, this volume is estimated to be 150 ml for the so-called "average man." DSA might be considered stagnant, because it never reaches the alveoli, nor is it completely flushed out during expiration. Consequently, it does not contribute to effective ventilation of the alveoli. Its volume must be deducted from the tidal volume per breath to arrive at a value for alveolar ventilation. In terms of the preceding example, the runner's ventilatory requirement of 20 ℓ/min. could be satisfied, on the one hand, by an increase in f only, as follows:

$$\dot{V}_E = V_T \times f$$
$$= 0.500 \times 40 = 20 \text{ ℓ/min.}$$
$$\dot{V}_A = (V_T - DSA) \times f$$
$$= (0.500 - 0.150) \times 40$$
$$= 0.350 \times 40$$
$$= 14 \text{ ℓ/min.}$$

On the other hand, the requirement could be met by an increase in V_T only, as follows:

$$\dot{V}_E = V_T \times f$$
$$= 2.000 \times 10 = 20 \text{ ℓ/min.}$$

$$\dot{V}_A = (V_T - DSA) \times f$$
$$= (2.000 - 0.150) \times 10$$
$$= 1.850 \times 10$$
$$= 18.5 \, \ell/min.$$

From this example, it should be clear that alveolar ventilation is enhanced more by an increase in tidal volume than by an increase in frequency. While this holds true for most submaximal levels of work, there is a point at which the metabolic cost of deep breathing outweighs its advantage. At any rate, it appears helpful to consciously attempt to increase tidal volume to satisfy greater ventilatory demands during submaximal work. Many distance runners advocate that this increase in tidal volume be accomplished by "belly breathing," which they claim is more efficient than intercostal (chest) breathing.

REFERENCES

1. Astrand, P.O., and Rodahl, K. *Textbook of work physiology.* 2d ed. New York: McGraw-Hill, 1977.
2. Comroe, J.H. *Physiology of respiration.* Chicago: Yearbook Medical Publishers, 1965.
3. Guyton, A.C. *Textbook of medical physiology.* 5th ed. Philadelphia: W.B. Saunders, 1977.
4. Slonim, N.B., and Hamilton, L.H. *Respiratory physiology.* 2d ed. St. Louis: C.V. Mosby, 1971.

KEY TERMS
All-or-none law (p. 132)
Body alignment (p. 140)
Center of gravity (p. 137)
Force application (p. 138)
Force arm (p. 139)
Kinesthetic perception (p. 137)
Motor unit (p. 135)
Muscle fiber (p. 132)
Myofibrils (p. 133)
Posture (p. 140)
Resistance application (p. 138)
Resistance arm (p. 139)
Sarcolemma (p. 133)
Sarcoplasm (p. 133)
Stability (p. 137)

BEHAVIORAL OBJECTIVES
Upon completion of this chapter, the student should be able to:

1. Define the key terms listed above.
2. Describe the characteristics of skeletal, smooth, and cardiac muscle tissue.
3. Identify and describe the components of the gross structure of skeletal muscle.
4. Diagram a skeletal muscle fiber; define the *sacromere, actin* and *myosin filaments, Z-line, H-zone, A-band,* and *I-band* and identify these structures.
5. Describe the sliding-filament theory and the role of adenosine triphosphate (ATP).
6. Identify the factors responsible for gradation of muscular contraction.
7. List and define the types of muscular contraction.
8. Define the *principles of reciprocal innervation, equilibrium,* and *levers*; describe the relationship and importance of these principles to movement skills.
9. Describe the three classes of levers; state one mechanical example for each class and one anatomical example for first-class and third-class levers.
10. Describe good posture and movement mechanics for standing, walking, running for speed, running for distance, sitting, lifting, carrying heavy objects, and lying.

CHAPTER TEN

THE MUSCULAR SYSTEM, POSTURE, AND MOVEMENT MECHANICS

People cannot do anything without using some muscle, or muscles, as all movement and body functions depend upon the contraction of muscle tissue. There are three types of muscle tissue in the human body — skeletal, smooth, and cardiac.

Skeletal, striated muscle performs the functions of moving and stabilizing the skeletal system. It is innervated by the voluntary (somatic) nervous system and consists of long, cylindrical **muscle fibers**. Each fiber, or cell, has several hundred nuclei and is structurally independent of other fibers. Skeletal muscle is called *striated* because of its parallel layers of alternating light and dark bands.

Smooth, nonstriated muscle is found in the walls of the hollow *viscera* and blood vessels. It is innervated by the involuntary (autonomic) nervous system and ordinarily is not under voluntary control. Smooth muscle consists of long, spindle-shaped cells, and each cell usually has only one nucleus.

Cardiac muscle, the heart muscle, is a network of striated fibers interwoven to form a network called a *syncytium*. This arrangement of the fibers enables the cardiac muscle to contract as a unit, obeying the **all-or-none law.** Cardiac muscle also contracts rhythmically and automatically, as the impulse for contraction originates within the heart itself.

GROSS STRUCTURE OF SKELETAL MUSCLE

Skeletal muscle has an outside covering of connective tissue called the *epimysium*, which merges at the ends of the muscle with a tendon. The tendon connects the muscle to a bone.

Within a muscle, the fibers are grouped into bundles, referred to as *fasciculi*, which are covered by a connective tissue called the *perimysium*. The fasciculi vary in length and ordinarily do not run the full length of a large muscle. A fasciculus may have only a few muscle fibers or as many as 150 or more. (See Figure 10-1.)

MICROSCOPIC STRUCTURE OF SKELETAL MUSCLE

Each fiber is surrounded by a connective tissue, the *endomysium*. One fiber rarely runs the entire length of a muscle or even of a fasciculus. Hence the connective tissue of a muscle is necessary for the transmission of the force of contraction from one fiber to another, from the fibers to a fasciculus, from one fasciculus to another, and from the fasciculi to the tendon or tendons connected to the bone.

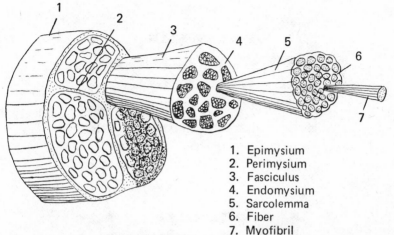

1. Epimysium
2. Perimysium
3. Fasciculus
4. Endomysium
5. Sarcolemma
6. Fiber
7. Myofibril

Figure 10-1. Construction of a skeletal muscle.

The smallest fibers cannot be seen with the naked eye, and the largest are as thick as a human hair. They vary in length, ranging from 1 to 50 mm, which in some cases is the entire length of the muscle.

Beneath the endomysium, the muscle cell is covered by a tough, exceedingly thin, elastic sheath, the **sarcolemma**, and beneath it are located the numerous nuclei. Embedded in the muscle-fiber protoplasm (**sarcoplasm**) are columnlike structures called **myofibrils**. (It is the myofibrils, with alternating segments of light and dark color, that impart the striated appearance to skeletal muscle.) They serve as the contractile units of the muscle. Each myofibril is subdivided into *sarcomeres*. These are the functional units of the myofibrils and are composed of two types of protein in parallel filaments. The thick filaments contain *myosin*, and the thin ones contain *actin.*

As shown in Figure 10-2, the thin filaments of actin form a light zone, called the *I-band*, and the thick myosin filaments form the denser, darker *A-band*. The actin filaments arise from a membrane called the *Z-line*, which forms the boundary between the sarcomeres. The spaces between pairs of actin filaments form a lighter band within the A-band, called the *H-zone.*

THE CONTRACTILE PROCESS

The most widely accepted explanation of muscle contraction is the *sliding-filament theory.* It contends that the actin filaments slide between the myosin filaments, which pulls the Z-lines of the sarcomere

Figure 10-2. Structure of a sarcomere.

toward the A-band and shortens the I-band. The length of the A-band is not changed; that is, the myosin filaments remain constant in length. However, the H-zone disappears in the sliding process. (See Figure 10-2.) The exact manner in which this process occurs is not completely understood, but it is believed that cross-bridges from the myosin filaments form a chemical bond with selected sites on the actin filaments.

Energy for muscle contraction is derived from the breakdown of *adenosine triphosphate (ATP)*. Nerve impulses sent to the muscle cell stimulate this breakdown, and the energy yielded is utilized when the actin filaments slide between the myosin filaments. The liberation of energy occurs in the following reaction: ATP = *adenosine diphosphate (ADP)* + phosphate + energy. ATP for further contraction is synthesized from nutrient substances and creatine phosphate. The latter, which is found only in muscle tissue, is broken down by enzymatic activity during exercise; its by-products combine with ADP to form ATP:

$$\text{creatine phosphate} \underset{}{\overset{\text{enzyme}}{\rightleftarrows}} \text{creatine} + \text{phosphates} + \text{energy}$$

$$\text{phosphates} + \text{energy} + \text{ADP} \rightleftarrows \text{ATP}$$

THE MOTOR UNIT

The basic unit of muscular contraction is the **motor unit**, which consists of a group of muscle cells innervated by the fiber of a single nerve cell. Upon entering the muscle through the epimysium, the nerve fiber branches and distributes itself among the muscle cells. The need for this arrangement can be seen in the huge difference that exists between the number of *motor nerves* entering a muscle and the number of muscle fibers (cells) within the muscle: there are about 250,000,000 separate muscle fibers that make up the human skeletal muscles, but there are only approximately 420,000 motor nerves (4). As every muscle fiber must be innervated, it is necessary that nerve fibers branch repeatedly.

The number of muscle fibers in a motor unit varies from muscle to muscle, in relation to the function of the muscle. Those performing fine and delicate work, such as the eye muscles, may have ratios of 1 nerve fiber to 5 or fewer muscle fibers, but muscles used for heavy work may have 150 or more muscle fibers per motor unit.

THE ALL-OR-NONE LAW

A muscle rarely contracts maximally as a whole, but a single fiber can only contract maximally. Upon receiving a stimulus of threshold value from a nerve fiber or its branch, an individual muscle fiber contracts completely or not at all. Since a single nerve cell supplies many muscle fibers in the formation of a motor unit, it is evident that the motor unit also functionally follows the all-or-none law.

The contraction force of the entire muscle varies in relation to a given set of conditions at the time of contraction. If appropriate nutrients are available and the muscle is warm and is not fatigued, the contraction can be strong. However, a weak contraction results if the muscle is cold and fatigued and the needed nutrients are not present.

MUSCLE FATIGUE

Fatigue occurs when the contractile and metabolic processes of muscle fibers are no longer able to continue a set work rate. Exercise physiologists do not agree upon what is the site of muscular fatigue. Its causes may include changes in the chemical properties of the muscle fibers, breakdown of the ATP/ADP system, depletion of the glycogen stores, and inability to remove the end products that accumulate during anaerobic work.

GRADATION OF MUSCULAR CONTRACTION

The strength, or gradation, of contraction is determined not by the individual motor unit but by two other factors. One is the number of motor units stimulated. A muscle might contain hundreds of motor units and, although all the fibers of a single motor unit must contract together, the many motor units of one muscle do not have to contract simultaneously. The size of the work load is evaluated by the cortex, and it stimulates an appropriate number of motor units. Sometimes an incorrect judgment is made, and more motor units are stimulated than are needed, as happens when one lifts an empty box that was believed to contain a heavy load. Conversely, too few motor units are stimulated when one first lifts a heavy box that was believed to be light.

The second factor in the gradation of muscular response is the frequency of stimulation, or the number of times per second that each motor unit is stimulated. A high-frequency succession of stimuli gives rise to a cumulative effect; this process is referred to as a *summation* of stimuli. The summation of contraction occurs when a second stimulus is initiated at the apex of the preceding one, so that the total tension of the muscle is increased.

TYPES OF CONTRACTION

Muscular contraction can result in shortening, maintaining a static position, or lengthening. Examples of these types of contraction follow.

During *isotonic contraction*, the muscle changes in length while a constant tension is applied to it. Shortening of the sarcomeres and movement take place. Push-ups, work with weights, and sit-ups require this type of contraction. *Dynamic* and *concentric contraction* are other names for isotonic contraction.

If a muscle remains a constant length during contraction, *isometric,* or *static, contraction* takes place. Pushing and pulling against an immovable object produce isometric contraction.

The gradual lengthening of a muscle from a shortened position is *eccentric contraction.* The triceps undergo eccentric contraction when they return to the down position during push-ups, as do the biceps brachii when the body is slowly lowered during chin-ups.

All three types of contraction have been used to increase strength; however, each has recognized advantages and disadvantages. Training regimens employing these types of contraction are discussed in greater detail in Chapter 4.

MECHANICAL PRINCIPLES

At rest or in motion, people must apply certain mechanical principles if general efficiency, reduction of energy expenditure, and improvement of physical performance are to take place. No attempt will be made here to state all of these principles, but *reciprocal innervation, equilibrium,* and *levers* will be discussed.

Reciprocal Innervation

For coordinated and graceful movement to occur, the muscles opposite the contracting muscles must be able to relax and lengthen easily. All muscles must also be able to contract strongly and quickly (5).

The ability to feel this contraction and relaxation, to know what a muscle is doing, to know the position of body parts, is **kinesthetic perception.** An individual who fails to develop this ability has no basis for feeling and sensing whether a movement is right or wrong and no basis for correcting an error in movement or for establishing a movement pattern. Kinesthetic perception develops as one consciously places the body or its parts in a position and "gets the feel" of that position. With practice, this ability to feel becomes habitual and serves as an important force for increasing the efficiency of movement (5).

Equilibrium

Equilibrium involves balance, **stability**, position, and stance. There can be various stages of stability, but the **center of gravity** is involved in all considerations of equilibrium. The center of gravity is the weight center of a body, the imaginary point at which all the body's parts exactly balance one another. For the human body, its location depends upon the individual's anatomic structure, posture, and position. If an individual of average build stands erect with the arms hanging at the sides, the center of gravity is located in the pelvis, in front of the upper sacrum. A female's center of gravity is usually lower than a male's because of her heavier pelvis and thighs and her shorter legs. In addition, the center of gravity can be shifted by a change in posture or a movement of the limbs and also by external weights that the body supports.

The ability to maintain stability under unfavorable conditions is a basic motor skill. Stability is affected by all of the following factors (3).
1.   Stability is directly proportional to the area of the base on which the body rests. An individual standing erect with the feet spread

about 12 to 14 in. apart is in a more stable position than one who stands with the feet very close together. Positions that place both hands and knees or feet on the ground establish a wider base and hence greater stability.

2. Stability in a given direction is directly proportional to the horizontal distance from the center of gravity to the edge of the support base in the direction of movement. A sprinter on the starting line leans forward so that the center of gravity is directly above the hands. This position creates a tendency to fall forward, which enables the runner to start quicker than someone whose center of gravity is over the feet.

3. Stability is directly proportional to the weight of the body. If two individuals assume postures with the same base of support, it is more difficult to move the heavier individual.

4. Stability is inversely proportional to the distance from the body's center of gravity to the base of support. The closer the center of gravity to the base of support, the greater the stability.

5. For equilibrium to exist, a vertical line through the body's center of gravity must fall within the base of support. If the center of gravity moves outside the base, the individual becomes less stable and more likely to fall. To perform a handstand, for example, the individual must maintain the center of gravity directly over the area between the hands.

Principle of Levers

A lever is a rigid bar that turns about a fixed point or an axis by the application of an external force. The purpose of a lever is to gain mechanical advantage, so that a small force can overcome a larger resistance. In the body, the bones serve as levers, and muscle contractions produce the forces that operate them. The resistances to motion can be internal or external or both (6).

The classification and effectiveness of a lever is dependent upon the location of three points: the fulcrum (axis), the point of **force application**, and the point of **resistance application.** If the fulcrum is located between the force and the resistance, it is designated a *first-class lever,* which is the most efficient kind. A teeter board and a scissors are mechanical first-class levers; the extension of the forearm by the triceps muscle and the flexion and extension of the head are anatomical first-class levers.

If the resistance is located between the fulcrum and the force, it is designated a *second-class lever.* A wheelbarrow is one example.

First-class lever

Second-class lever

Third-class lever

Figure 10-3. Three classes of levers.

Whether or not there are any second-class levers in the body appears to be a controversial matter among anatomists and kinesiologists (7).

In a *third-class lever*, the force is located between the fulcrum and the resistance. A door that is closed by a spring is a mechanical third-class lever; the flexion of the forearm by the biceps muscle is an anatomical third-class lever. Most of the body's movements are produced by this type.

The distance from the fulcrum to the force point is known as the **force arm**, and the distance from the fulcrum to the resistance point is known as the **resistance arm**. The relative lengths of the two arms determine the way the lever functions. A first-class lever is built for equilibrium, a second-class one for reduction of force, and a third-class one for speed and range of movement (6). In anatomical levers, the force arm is comparatively short, so that muscle contraction provides a relatively weak force, but this arrangement enables that force to move the resistance quickly. Thus it is possible to run, jump, and throw with great velocity, but it is difficult to life a heavy weight with a third-class lever.

The arrangement of the body's leverage system causes the joints to be very susceptible to injury, and individuals participating in contact sports, such as football, often suffer damage to the shoulders, knees, and ankles.

POSTURE AND MOVEMENT MECHANICS

For efficient movement to take place, correct **posture (body alignment)** is mandatory. The postures that are maintained for various positions and movements are the result of conscious and unconscious practice, which usually leads to the formation of postural habits. They may be good habits, which contribute to attractive appearance and to mechanical efficiency, or they may be poor habits, which contribute to incorrect muscle development, tension, spinal deviations, lower back disorders, poor circulation, and unattractive appearance.

Postural habits are developed as the individual repeatedly assumes a given body alignment during work, play, and relaxation. While one is in this position, a response is established in the neuromuscular system. This response becomes habitual, so that it is produced even though the individual is unconscious of posture. The habitual postural response occurs whether the habit is good or bad, and many individuals mistakenly feel comfortable in a position that actually places a strain on the joints (5).

The habits of poor posture cannot be overcome with a few minutes of daily exercise. The neuromuscular system must be given thorough reeducation over an extended period of time to establish good body alignment and mechanics.

In summary, Metheny (5) describes the following conditions as fundamental for the development of effective posture and movement: (1) every muscle should have sufficient strength and tone to perform its functions; (2) every muscle should have sufficient relaxation to perform its functions easily; (3) the joints should have flexibility that provides for a full range of movement; (4) kinesthetic perception should be highly developed; and (5) good posture development should be continuous throughout the day and should be controlled to produce the best results in strength, relaxation, flexibility, and efficiency of movement.

These conditions can be met by an individual who has (1) a knowledge of the movement process and the mechanics of efficient movement, (2) the ability to control his or her neuromuscular system, and (3) the desire to acquire an effective posture (5). The following mechanical descriptions are listed to provide the knowledge necessary for an individual to experience efficient posture and movement.

Standing (8)

1. The head and chin are centered over the trunk and are held in a relaxed position at right angles to the front of the neck.
2. The shoulders are free and easy and are neither forward, back, nor elevated.
3. The shoulder blades are drawn down and flat on the back.
4. The chest is held up and is neither sagging nor too high nor leading.
5. The trunk is within normal limits of curves, neither too straight and flat nor too round and hollow.
6. The abdomen is up and in and is neither relaxed nor protruding.
7. The hips are in line with the trunk and are neither leading nor thrust back.
8. The arms hang naturally and relaxed at the sides and are neither held rigidly nor too relaxed.
9. The knees are free and easy and are neither bent nor thrust back.
10. The feet are parallel and slightly apart.
11. The weight falls ahead of the outer anklebone and is distributed toward the outside of each foot.

From the front view of this position, the weight should be evenly distributed about a vertical line through the midpoint of the body. From the side view, a vertical line should pass through the earlobe, through the middle of the shoulder and the middle of the hip, slightly behind the kneecap, and slightly in front of the outer anklebone. The center of gravity should be directly over the base of support.

Walking (5)

1. The upper body (head, chin, shoulders, and chest) should be balanced on the trunk; it should not be dragged forward by the pull of gravity.
2. The trunk should be balanced in the pelvic basin; it does not come to an erect, rigid position between steps, but remains inclined slightly forward to keep it in line with the extended rear leg at the time of the push-off. The center of gravity should not be carried beyond the base of support.

3. Motion should originate in the hip joint as the leading leg is swung ahead of the body.
4. The leading leg is always parallel to or in advance of the trunk, so that a new base of support is always ready to receive the body weight.
5. As a new base of support is established, the upper body remains in line with the axis of the rear leg.
6. The supporting and pushing leg applies its force directly through the center of gravity along the line of resistance of the trunk. This leg begins to push off before the front foot strikes the ground.
7. The heel strikes the ground first, directly in line with the direction of walk. The weight is transferred through the outer border of the foot to the ball of the foot.
8. The ankle joint is extended as the final push or thrust is made with the big toe.
9. The weight shift to the alternate foot causes the pelvic girdle to oscillate back and forth. The arms and shoulders swing slightly to compensate for this oscillation and to keep the body weight evenly distributed.
10. The leg muscles should supply most of the energy for locomotion, so that the body makes as few extraneous motions as possible.

Running for Speed (2, 3)

1. The trunk should be upright to keep the runner in balance. Leaning forward places the body off balance, which forces the leg muscles to exert additional effort to prevent a fall. With the trunk upright, the center of gravity can be forward of the pushing foot.
2. As a long lever develops more speed at the end than does a short lever, the lead leg should be fully extended at the moment of the push from the rear leg. This action also enables the full force of the push to be converted into forward movement.
3. Any vertical movement should be just great enough to counteract the downward pull of gravity but not great enough to produce an unnecessary bounce, since the foward speed of the runner is decreasing while the body is off the ground. The higher the center of gravity rises, the longer the body is off the ground.
4. As the foot leaves the ground after a vigorous push, the knee is bent. The faster the leg moves, the more the knee is bent, and the higher the foot is raised. By this action, the knee moves forward with greater angular velocity due to the shorter radius of the arc through which the leg swings.
5. The faster one moves, the higher the knee should be raised in

front. This movement delays the placing of the foot on the ground for its next thrust and permits the lead leg to reach full extension.

6. The runner should alight on the ball of the foot.
7. The faster one runs, the longer the stride. However, if the stride is too long, the runner's foot contacts the ground ahead of the center of gravity, which produces a braking action.
8. The swing of the arms should be coordinated with that of the legs in order to balance the rotary effect of the leg swing on the trunk.

Running for Distance (1)

1. The head should remain up to avoid the tendency to watch the feet.
2. The back should be straight but naturally comfortable. Do not throw back the shoulders and stick out the chest.
3. The buttocks should be "tucked in." In this position, a hypothetical line drawn through the shoulders and the hips should be vertical or nearly so.
4. The elbows are bent and held slightly away from the body. One should avoid placing them out like wings or pressing them to the chest; they should not be carried at hip or belt level.
5. The body should be straight as the legs move freely from the hips. The legs should be lifted from the knees while the ankles are relaxed. The runner should not overstride; each foot should fall just under the knee.
6. Using the heel-to-toe method for footstrike, one should land on the heel, then rock forward to take off from the ball of the foot. This method is the least tiring over long distances and is the least wearing, as the heel cushions the landing and the forward rocking distributes the pressure.
7. In the flat-foot method for footstrike, the foot falls under the knee in a quick, light action with the entire foot landing on the ground at the same time. This type of landing provides a wide surface area to cushion the footstrike. The foot should not be driven down but should be allowed to pass beneath the body.

Sitting (5)

1. The head, neck, and shoulders should be in the same position as for standing.
2. The back of the buttocks should touch the back of the chair. All the support of the chair should be used.
3. The feet should be flat on the floor. There may be variations in the position of the legs and feet, but the hips should remain toward the back of the chair.

4. If one writes or reads while sitting at a table, the chair should be brought well under the table, so that the edge of the table almost touches the front of the body. Sit all the way back in the chair and allow the trunk to slant forward slightly from the hip joint to bring the eyes in line with the work. Keep the head-neck-trunk line as straight as possible for maximum support of the head.

Lifting Heavy Objects

1. The knees should be bent and the back should remain straight.
2. The feet should be spread apart about shoulder width.
3. The lifting should be performed by straightening the legs.

Carrying Heavy Objects

1. The center of gravity should always be above the base of support.
2. The body alignment should be altered as little as possible.
3. The object should be carried as close to the body's center of gravity as possible and no higher than waist level.

Lying

1. If one is lying on the back, a pillow should be placed under the knees to help prevent exaggerated curvature of the lower back. The head should be elevated only slightly.
2. If one is lying on the side, both knees should be drawn up to relieve lower back strain.
3. If one is lying on the stomach, a pillow should be placed under the stomach and hips to help keep the back straight.

REFERENCES

1. Bowerman, W.J., and Harris, W.D. *Jogging.* New York: Grosset and Dunlap, 1967.
2. Broer, M.R. *Efficiency of human movement.* 3d ed. Philadelphia: W.B. Saunders, 1973.
3. Bunn, J.W. *Scientific principles of coaching.* Englewood Cliffs: Prentice-Hall, 1955.
4. Mathews, D.K., and Fox, E.L. *The physiological basis of physical education and athletics.* 2d ed. Philadelphia: W.B. Saunders, 1976.
5. Metheny, E. *Body dynamics.* New York: McGraw-Hill, 1952.
6. Scott, M.G. *Analysis of human motion.* 2d ed. New York: Appleton-Century-Crofts, 1963.
7. Wells, K.F. *Kinesiology.* Philadelphia: W.B. Saunders, 1971.
8. Wessel, J. *Movement fundamentals.* 2d ed. Englewood Cliffs: Prentice-Hall, 1961.

In this book, the authors have attempted to provide the reader with information concerning human response to a regular exercise program (training), the benefits as well as the risks associated with engagement in such a program, and some of the biological and psychological consequences of failure to remain physically active throughout life. Exposure to this information should convince the reader to make a commitment to a lifetime exercise program.

This program should be based on sound scientific principles and should be developed to meet the needs of each particular individual. A summary of these principles and the procedures for development of an exercise program are provided below.

For individuals under age 35 with no previous history of cardiovascular disease and without any of the CHD primary risk factors, no medical clearance is required prior to participation in a physical exercise program. All individuals above age 35 are advised to receive medical clearance before they begin training.

Once the individual has determined that there are no contraindications to an exercise program, either a graded exercise test or a self-evaluation technique for circulorespiratory endurance should be administered. A physical exercise program can then be planned with consideration given to (1) the type of exercise to be conducted, (2) the frequency of training, and (3) the desired intensity and duration of each work period.

The type of exercise program is dictated by the particular components of physical fitness that the individual wishes to develop or maintain—circulorespiratory endurance, muscular endurance and strength, flexibility, and weight management. Ideally, a regular exercise program would emphasize all these components. However, if an individual cannot devote enough time and effort to pursue an all-encompassing program, the com-

145

ponents of circulorespiratory endurance, flexibility, and weight management should take precedence.

Circulorespiratory endurance is developed through aerobic activities, e.g., running, walking, swimming, or cycling for a relatively long distance or jumping rope for an extended period of time. The individual should select an aerobic activity or activities that he or she enjoys performing and one to which he or she can make a commitment to continue. Running is the best aerobic activity for development and maintenance of circulorespiratory endurance, but some individuals find it boring. In addition, individuals with joint problems (in the back, knees, and ankles) and feet disorders are unable to run for an extended period of time. Aside from the other activities just mentioned, singles play in tennis, racquetball, or handball is an excellent alternative to running if the participants have enough skill to produce continuous play or rallies. Unless both players have a moderate degree of skill, there usually is not enough movement in these sports to develop circulorespiratory endurance. Sports such as golf and bowling definitely do not require sufficient physical intensity to achieve that objective.

An exercise program designed to develop circulorespiratory endurance should be performed a minimum of three (nonconsecutive) days per week; however, a daily program is preferable. Many individuals exercise five to seven days per week but prefer to modify the intensity or the duration or both on alternate days, e.g., they exercise with greater intensity and for a longer period of time every other day, or three or four days per week.

Determining the intensity at which one should exercise is difficult, but, if training effects are to occur, the principle of overload must be observed. Sedentary individuals who initiate an exercise program should begin at a relatively low intensity and gradually increase the level of exertion. Many individuals undertake a program with great expectations of physical development, but they mistakenly begin their activity at an intensity that is too high for them. Their efforts result in soreness and discomfort, which hinder continuation of the program, and, upon recovery from the soreness, these individuals have no desire to resume.

Monitoring the heart rate is the easiest method to determine the intensity at which one is working. Unless advised differently by a qualified physician, one should exercise at a minimum of 60% of one's maximum heart range. As the level of circulorespiratory endurance increases, this percentage can be increased. The heart rate can be used to indicate the intensity of all aerobic activities.

The duration of each exercise period is determined by the objectives of the program. The individual should devote 5 to 10 minutes to flexibility exercises and a minimum of 15 minutes to aerobic activity. As the level of circulorespiratory endurance improves, the duration of the exercise period can and perhaps should be increased.

It is well known that flexibility is specific to particular joints and to particular sports and that it decreases during the aging process; therefore, the individual should maintain a flexibility program for the entire body, with special emphasis on neck and shoulder flexibility, back extension, hip flexion, and posterior leg extension. Participants in a regular exercise program should be aware that many aerobic activities do not contribute to flexibility and, in fact, can actually decrease it; for example, jogging decreases the flexibility of the posterior upper and lower leg muscles. For all these reasons, static stretching daily or at least five days per week is recommended. In addition, sets of stretching for each specific flexibility should be performed several times throughout the day rather than all at once.

Weight management involves a combination of diet and exercise, as caloric intake must be balanced by caloric expenditure (energy needs). It has been demonstrated that a combination of decreased caloric intake and increased physical activity is the most effective procedure for weight loss. The distance one walks, runs, cycles, or swims, rather than the intensity of performance, is important for weight loss. The same number of calories is utilized whether one walks or runs for a specified distance. For effective development of circulo-respiratory endurance and weight management, one should consider both the intensity and the duration of the exercise program.

Participation in a regular exercise program must be based on a personal decision. Excuses that are often given for not doing so — lack of time, of facilities, of motivation — should be reexamined in relation to the benefits of such a program. To enhance the quality of life, everyone should make regular, vigorous exercise a lifetime commitment.

APPENDIX
(COOPER'S TWELVE-MINUTE RUN)

Cooper's Twelve-Minute Run is a test of cardiorespiratory function. It should be performed *only* after the safety precautions (contraindications to exercise) described in Chapter 3 have been read.

The object of the test is to run, jog, or walk as far as possible during a 12-minute period. The distance is measured either in miles or in laps around the perimeter of a 94-ft. by 50-ft. rectangle. One lap equals 288 ft. It is calculated that an additional 12 ft. are added where the runner turns the four corners, so that one lap is actually at least 300 ft.

For a complete set of instructions for the test, see Laboratory Session 5.

Table A-1 converts laps to miles and assigns fitness categories based on the test. Table A-2 lists percentile scores for the test.

TABLE A-1
FITNESS CATEGORIES BASED ON COOPER'S TWELVE-MINUTE RUN

Category	Laps*	Miles	$\dot{V}O_2$ (in ml/kg/min.)[†]
Men			
Excellent	30.8 or more	1.75 or more	51.6 or greater
Good	26.4-30.7	1.50-1.74	42.6-51.5
Fair	22.0-26.3	1.25-1.49	33.8-42.5
Poor	21.9 or fewer	1.24 or fewer	33.7 or less
Women			
Excellent	29.0 or more	1.65 or more	. . . .
Good	23.8-28.9	1.35-1.64	. . . .
Fair	20.2-23.7	1.15-1.34	. . . .
Poor	20.1 or fewer	1.14 or fewer	. . . .

SOURCE: Kenneth H. Cooper, *The new aerobics* (New York: M. Evans, 1970).

* Assuming 17.6 laps per mile.

[†] No data available for women.

TABLE A-2
PERCENTILE SCORES FOR COOPER'S 12-MINUTE RUN

Men			Women		
Laps	*Yards*	*%tile*	*Laps*	*Yards*	*%tile*
35	3500	100.0	28	2800	100.0
34	3400	97.5	27	2700	97.0
33	3300	95.0	26	2600	94.0
32	3200	92.5	25	2500	91.0
31	3100	90.0	24	2400	88.0
30	3000	87.5	23	2300	85.0
29	2900	85.0	22	2200	82.0
28	2800	82.5	21	2100	79.0
27	2700	80.0	20	2000	76.0
26	2600	77.5	19	1900	73.0
25	2500	75.0	18	1800	70.0
24	2400	72.5	17	1700	67.0
23	2300	70.0	16	1600	64.0
22	2200	67.5	15	1500	61.0
21	2100	65.0			
20	2000	62.5			
19	1900	60.0			

NOTE: These scores are developed for indoor administration of the test with laps around a standard basketball court (94 ft. x 50 ft.).

GLOSSARY

Adenosine Diphosphate. A compound (ester) composed of one molecule each of adenine and D-ribose and two molecules of phosphoric acid. It is formed as a result of the breakdown of adenosine triphosphate and is used in the resynthesis of adenosine triphosphate.

Adenosine triphosphate. A compound (ester) composed of one molecule each of adenine and D-ribose and three molecules of phosphoric acid. Its breakdown by hydrolysis is accompanied by the release of energy for muscular and other types of cellular activity.

Adrenal glands. Endocrine glands, one located immediately above each kidney. They produce epinephrine and norepinephrine and many steroidal hormones involved in electrolyte and fluid balance.

Aerobic power (aerobic capacity). The capacity of one's heart, lungs, and vascular system to deliver oxygen to working muscles.

Asymptomatic. Presenting none of the symptoms usually connected with the identification of particular diseases.

Baroreceptors. Nerve endings in various arteries that respond to pressure (e.g., blood pressure, stretching, touching).

Beriberi. A disease caused by deficiency of thiamine (vitamin B_1). It is characterized by cardiovascular abnormalities, edema, and cerebral manifestations and other nerve damage.

Body image. The feelings and attitudes an individual has towards his or her body.

Catecholamines. One of a group of similar compounds that mimic responses to activity of the sympathetic nervous system. Examples are epinephrine and norepinephrine.

Collateral circulation. Circulation through extra blood vessels that supply additional blood to specific areas of the body. It provides alternative routes in case of occlusion of an artery. It develops naturally if the opening in an artery becomes critically small.

Distributed practice. A system of practice schedules that are separated by either rest or some activity that is different from the one being practiced.

Dynamic contraction. Isotonic contraction: a type of muscle contraction in which shortening of the muscle fibers occurs. Movement is involved.

Eccentric contraction. A type of muscle contraction in which there is a gradual lengthening of the muscle fibers from a shortened position against resistance.

Extracellular fluid. Fluid that is found outside of the cells of the body.

Fibrinolysis. The activity of the fibrinolysin system, which removes small clots from tiny vessels throughout the body.

Glucose. A simple sugar belonging to the monosaccharide group, which is oxidized in the body to liberate heat and energy.

Glycogen. Animal starch, which is stored in the animal body for future conversion into sugar (glucose) and for subsequent use as a source of energy.

Hemodynamic. Related to circulation or to the cardiovascular system.

Histological. Pertaining to structure.

Homeostatic balance. The presence of physiological equilibrium in which body functions and conditions are within an acceptable and safe range.

Hyperextension. Extreme extension or overextension of a joint of the body.

Hypokinetic disease. Malady due to lack of movement.

Interventricular septum. Tissue that separates the left side of the heart from the right side.

Intracellular fluid. Fluid that is found within the cell wall.

Isokinetic contraction. A type of muscular contraction in which the speed of the contraction and the resistance encountered are unchanged during the entire range of motion.

Isometric contraction. Static contraction: a type of muscle contraction in which no shortening of the muscle fibers occurs, which thus produces no movement.

Isotonic contraction. See **Dynamic contraction.**

IU. International unit, a quantity of a substance (e.g., a vitamin) that produces a particular biological effect agreed upon as an international standard.

Lactacid. The portion of an oxygen debt in which lactic acid is accumulated. This portion is repaid very slowly.

Lactic acid. A by-product of anaerobic metabolism which results from the incomplete oxidation of glucose during muscular work. It is capable of terminating muscular contraction if its concentration is high enough.

Lesion. Any pathological or traumatic discontinuity of tissue or loss of function of a part.

Lipid. Any one of a group of organic substances that are insoluble in water but soluble in alcohol, ether, chloroform, and other fat solvents. It has a greasy feel.

Massed practice. A system of practice schedules that have little or no rest or alternate activity between the beginning and the end of the activity being practiced.

MET. The metabolic equivalent of resting oxygen uptake expressed in terms of milliliters per kilogram of body weight per minute.

Metabolism. The sum of all the physical and chemical processes by which living organized substance is produced and maintained; also, the transformation by which energy is made available for the uses of an organism.

Motor Nerves. Fibers of tissue that conduct impulses from the brain to the muscle tissue. The impulse must be transmitted if movement is to take place.

Murmur (heart). One of various sounds produced by the heart during specific events of the cardiac cycle, usually the result of a leaky or narrowed valve. It may or may not be pathologic.

Neuritis. Inflammation of a nerve or nerves, which is marked by pain, sensory disturbances, and impaired reflexes.

Neuromuscular efficiency. Control of the muscles by the motor-nerve stimuli in the least wasteful manner.

Oxygen consumption. The amount of oxygen processed by the body. It is usually expressed in liters per minute but sometimes expressed in milliliters per kilogram of body weight per minute, to allow interpersonal comparisons to be made. Also called *oxygen intake* and *oxygen uptake*.

Oxygen extraction. The amount of oxygen extracted from 100 ml of blood.

Palpation. The act of feeling with the hand by light finger pressure.

Peripheral circulation. Blood flow through small vessels surrounded by muscles.

Peristalsis. Alternate contractions and relaxations of the smooth muscle of the esophagus, stomach, and intestines.

Pernicious anemia. A progressive decrease in the number and increase in the size of red blood cells, which results in weakness and gastrointestinal and nervous disturbances.

Relaxation. The relief or reduction of tension in the body. It reduces muscle tonus.

Repetition max (RM). The maximum number of times that one can repeat an exercise with a specified amount of weight.

Self-concept. An individual's perception of the kind of person he or she is.

Self-estimate. An individual's success or failure as defined by himself or herself.

Self-image. An individual's view of himself or herself at a particular time and place.

Static contraction. See **Isometric contraction.**

Stress. Any situation in which the body's homeostatic balance is disturbed.

Stressor. Any psychological or physical condition that disturbs the homeostatic balance of the body; anything that causes stress.

Stretch reflex. The reflex contraction of a muscle in response to being suddenly stretched beyond its normal length. This reflex action serves to prevent injury due to overstretching.

Sympathetic nervous system. A division of the autonomic, or involuntary, nervous system, which is responsible for promoting the body's reactions to a stressor.

Symptomatic. Presenting symptoms of a known condition, usually pathologic.

Tension. Increased muscle tonus, in which the muscles are contracted more than is necessary to maintain posture.

Viscera. Internal organs.

Work-relief ratio. The proportion between time spent working and time spent recovering. A work-relief ratio of 1:2 means that the recovery period is twice as long as the work period.

INDEX

KNOWLEDGE AND ATTITUDE ABOUT THE PURPOSE AND VALUE OF PHYSICAL ACTIVITY

Name _____   Instructor _____

Class and section _____   Date _____

Purpose

The purpose of this laboratory session is to evaluate your knowledge and attitude about the purpose and value of physical activity.

Equipment Needed

None

Procedure

Read each of the 45 items listed below and answer them yes or no. Give the answer that best indicates your knowledge or attitude.

Results

In today's society most individuals need to participate in a regular physical activity program, but many fail to do so due to their lack of knowledge about the value of physical fitness and their attitude toward physical activity. Observe how many questions you answered no. These answers may indicate a lack of knowledge about and a negative attitude toward physical activity.

Do you believe that an increased knowledge about the value of physical fitness and participation in a regular physical activity program can change a negative attitude toward physical activity?

Read each of the statements listed below and check either yes or no.

Yes   No

____   ____   1. Do you avoid the use of labor-saving devices whenever possible (e.g., riding lawn mowers and riding golf carts)?

Yes   No

_____   _____   2. Do you regularly perform work that requires vigorous physical exertion?

_____   _____   3. Do you regularly (at least three times per week) participate in physically active lifetime sports (e.g., tennis, racquetball, handball, or badminton)?

_____   _____   4. Do you regularly (at least three times per week) participate in aerobic activities that involve a minimum of 20 minutes of continuous movement (e.g., jogging, jumping rope, bicycling, or swimming)?

_____   _____   5. Do you believe that you can jog 2 mi. and continue your daily activities without experiencing fatigue in the evening?

_____   _____   6. Do you know the guidelines and precautions that should be followed when you first begin an exercise program?

_____   _____   7. Can you plan an exercise program for a 40-year-old sedentary individual?

_____   _____   8. Are you able to describe the benefits of a regular exercise program?

_____   _____   9. Are you able to estimate the energy expenditure of various physical activities?

_____   _____   10. Do you know the differences among circuit, interval, and aerobic training?

_____   _____   11. Are you able to develop an individualized training program for strength improvement?

_____   _____   12. Are you able to identify the primary and secondary risk factors associated with the development of coronary heart disease?

_____   _____   13. Are you able to identify safe ranges for blood pressure, serum cholesterol, and serum triglycerides?

_____   _____   14. Are you able to describe the role of exercise in the prevention of and the rehabilitation after coronary heart disease?

Yes　　No

15. Are you able to select and self-administer a suitable test for classification of the functional capacity of the circulorespiratory system?

16. Are you able to determine your target heart rate for training?

17. Are you able to state the physiological adaptations to endurance training and to strength training?

18. Are you able to develop an individualized training program for the improvement of circulorespiratory endurance?

19. Are you aware of the problems and disorders associated with the lack of flexibility?

20. Are you able to determine your flexibility in the neck, shoulder, chest, trunk, lower back, hips, and hamstring muscles?

21. Are you able to design an individualized program to develop flexibility?

22. Do you know the major reasons why individuals are overweight?

23. Do you know the effects of being overweight?

24. Do you know the difference between saturated and unsaturated fat?

25. Are you able to describe an adequate diet in relation to carbohydrate, protein, and fat percentages?

26. Are you able to describe a weight reduction plan in relation to caloric intake and exercise?

27. Do you know the characteristics of a tense individual?

28. Can you identify any stress-related diseases and disorders?

29. Can you describe the role of exercise in helping to prevent stress-related disorders?

Yes   No

_____ _____ 30. Are you able to release tension through a re- laxation technique?

_____ _____ 31. Are you able to state the maximal normal values for heart rate and systolic blood pressure?

_____ _____ 32. Are you able to describe the changes in respiratory function that result from long-term endurance training?

_____ _____ 33. Are you able to describe good posture and move- ment mechanics for standing, running for distance, lifting, and sitting?

_____ _____ 34. Do you avoid the use of alcohol and tranquilizers after a stressful experience or a bad day?

_____ _____ 35. Do you believe you have good eating habits?

_____ _____ 36. Are you able to relax immediately when you go to bed at night?

_____ _____ 37. Do you enjoy social interaction through participa- tion in sports?

_____ _____ 38. Do you have a socially acceptable way of releasing aggressive drives and hostile feelings?

_____ _____ 39. Is your typical day free from an unusual number of stressful experiences?

_____ _____ 40. Have you avoided any weight gain during the past year?

_____ _____ 41. Do you believe you have good posture when walking and sitting?

_____ _____ 42. Do you know the relationship of percentage of body fat and acceptable body weight?

_____ _____ 43. Do you like yourself?

_____ _____ 44. Do you enjoy mental and physical challenge?

_____ _____ 45. Are you physically fit?

LABORATORY 2
FLEXIBILITY EVALUATION

Name _____   Instructor _____

Class and section _____   Date _____

Purpose

The purpose of this laboratory session is to evaluate your flexibility in the neck, shoulders and shoulder girdle, chest muscles, trunk extension, trunk and hips, lower back and hips, and hamstring muscles.

Equipment Needed

1. Bench
2. Ruler or yardstick

Procedures

1. Take the flexibility tests described on pp. 50-53.
2. Record your scores in the Results section. Report the first three tests (shoulder lift, trunk extension, and sit and reach) in inches. Report the remaining four tests as passed (P) or failed (F).
3. Use Table 5-1 (p. 52) to determine your flexibility classification for the first three tests.

Results

Flexibility is not a general factor, but is specific to given joints and sports or physical activities. Active individuals tend to be more flexible than inactive individuals. Do you need to develop additional

flexibility? _____

Test	Score	Classification
Shoulder Lift (Fig. 5-1, p. 50)	____	_____
Trunk Extension (Fig. 5-2, p. 51)	____	_____
Sit and Reach (Fig. 5-3, p. 51)	____	_____
Neck Flexibility (Fig. 5-4, p. 52)	____	_____
Hips and Lower Back (Fig. 5-5, p. 52)	____	_____

Hamstring Muscles (Fig. 5-6, p. 53)   ____   _____

Chest Muscles (Fig. 5-7, p. 53)   ____   _____

LABORATORY 3
FLEXIBILITY EXERCISES

Name _____   Instructor _____

Class and section _____   Date _____

Purpose

The purposes of this laboratory session are:
1. To provide the opportunity to practice the flexibility exercises described on pp. 54-71.
2. To guide you in the formation of a flexibility program that can be conducted throughout your lifetime.

Equipment Needed

Towels

Procedures

Perform each of the flexibility exercises described on pp. 54-71. Follow all the instructions concerning duration and mechanics.

Results

1. Did you experience difficulty with any of the exercises? _____

2. Do you believe you should perform certain flexibility exercises daily? _____

3. What do you think will happen to your flexibility as you grow older? _____

It is impossible to state how much flexibility is desirable, but everyone should strive to prevent loss of flexibility, as the lack of it can create disorders or functional problems.

ESTIMATION OF
HEART ATTACK RISK

Name _____   Instructor _____

Class and section _____   Date _____

Purpose

The purpose of this laboratory session is to provide you with an estimate of your chances of suffering a heart attack now and in the future. You will make this estimate by playing the game RISKO.

Equipment Needed

1. Sphygmomanometer
2. Stethoscope
3. RISKO Game Card and Score Sheet

Procedure

1. Play the game as the directions indicate for your present age. (See pp. 168-170.)
2. Play the game a second time with data you estimate to be descriptive of your mother (for women) or your father (for men).

Results

1. What is your RISKO score? _____

2. What is your RISKO classification? _____

3. What is your parent's score? _____

4. What is your parent's classification? _____

5. List the factors that you might be able to change to decrease your chances of suffering a heart attack.

RISKO

The purpose of this game is to give you an estimate of your chances of suffering heart attack.

The game is played by marking squares which — from left to right — represent an increase in your risk factors. These are medical conditions and habits associated with an increased danger of heart attack. *Not all risk factors are measurable enough to be included in this game.*

Rules:

Study each risk factor and its row. Find the box applicable to you and circle the large number in it. For example, if you are 37, circle the number in the box labeled 31-40.

After checking out all the rows, add the circled numbers. This total — your score — is an estimate of your risk.

If you score:

6-11 — Risk well below average
12-17 — Risk below average
18-24 — Risk generally average
25-31 — Risk moderate
32-40 — Risk at a dangerous level
41-62 — Danger urgent. See your doctor now.

Heredity:

Count parents, grand-parents, brothers, and sisters who have had heart attack and/or stroke.

Tobacco smoking:

If you inhale deeply and smoke a cigarette way down, add one to your classification. Do not subtract because you think you do not inhale or smoke only a half inch on a cigarette.

Exercise:

Lower your score one point if you exercise regularly and frequently.

Cholesterol or saturated fat intake level:

A cholesterol blood test is best. If you can't get one from your doctor, then estimate honestly the percentage of solid fats you eat. These are usually of animal origin — lard, cream, butter, and beef and lamb fat. If you eat much of this, your cholesterol level probably will be high. The U.S. average, 40%, is too high for good health.

Blood pressure:

If you have no recent reading but have passed an insurance or industrial examination chances are you are 140 or less.

Sex:

This line takes into account the fact that men have from 6 to 10 times more heart attacks than women of child bearing age.

RISKO SCORE

Name _____ Sex _____ Date _____
Place the correct score for each factor on the appropriate line.

	Yourself	Dad or Mom
Age	_____	_____
Heredity	_____	_____
Weight	_____	_____
Tobacco smoking	_____	_____
Exercise	_____	_____
Cholesterol or fat percentage in diet	_____	_____
Blood pressure	_____	_____
Sex	_____	_____
Total	_____	_____
Classification	_____	_____

Factor						
Age	**1** 10 to 20	**2** 21 to 30	**3** 31 to 40	**4** 41 to 50	**6** 51 to 60	**8** 61 to 70 and over
Heredity	**1** No known history of heart disease	**2** 1 relative with cardiovascular disease Over 60	**3** 2 relatives with cardiovascular disease Over 60	**4** 1 relative with cardiovascular disease Under 60	**6** 2 relatives with cardiovascular disease Under 60	**8** 3 relatives with cardiovascular disease Under 60
Weight	**0** More than 5 lbs. below standard weight	**1** −5 to +5 lbs. standard weight	**2** 6-20 lbs. over weight	**3** 21-35 lbs. over weight	**5** 36-50 lbs. over weight	**7** 51-65 lbs. over weight
Tobacco smoking	**0** Non-user	**1** Cigar and/or pipe	**2** 10 cigarettes or less a day	**4** 20 cigarettes a day	**6** 30 cigarettes a day	**10** 40 cigarettes a day or more
Exercise	**1** Intensive occupational & recreational exertion	**2** Moderate occupational & recreational exertion	**3** Sedentary work & intense recreational exertion	**5** Sedentary occupational and moderate exertion	**6** Sedentary work & light recreational exertion	**8** Complete lack of all exercise
Cholesterol or fat % in diet	**1** Cholesterol below 180 mg%. Diet contains no animal or solid fats	**2** Cholesterol 181-205 mg%. Diet contains 10% animal or solid fats	**3** Cholesterol 206-230 mg%. Diet contains 20% animal or solid fats	**4** Cholesterol 231-255 mg%. Diet contains 30% animal or solid fats	**5** Cholesterol 256-280 mg%. Diet contains 40% animal or solid fats	**7** Cholesterol 281-300 mg%. Diet contains 50% animal or solid fats
Blood pressure	**1** 100 upper reading	**2** 120 upper reading	**3** 140 upper reading	**4** 160 upper reading	**6** 180 upper reading	**8** 200 or over upper reading
Sex	**1** Female under 40	**2** Female 40-50	**3** Female over 50	**4** Male	**6** Stocky male	**7** Bald stocky male

EVALUATION OF CIRCULORESPIRATORY FITNESS (COOPER'S TWELVE-MINUTE RUN)

Name _____   Instructor _____

Class and section _____   Date _____

Purpose

The purpose of this laboratory session is to evaluate your present level of circulorespiratory fitness by means of Cooper's Twelve-Minute Run. This test is based on research that demonstrates that the distance one can cover in 12 minutes correlates very highly with the ability of one's body to utilize large amounts of oxygen.

Equipment Needed

1. Timing device that will run for 12 minutes consecutively
2. Method of measuring the distance covered
   This can be counted in miles or in laps around a 94-ft. x 50-ft. rectangle. One lap equals 288 ft. It is calculated that an additional 12 ft. are added when a runner rounds off the four corners so that one lap is actually at least 300 ft.

Procedure

1. The object of the participant is to cover as much distance as possible in the allowed 12-minute period.
2. Start the timer, then run, jog, or walk for 12 consecutive minutes.
3. Determine the distance covered in miles.
4. Refer to Table A-1 (see p. 149) to find your fitness level.
5. Alternative procedure: Construct a rectangle 94 ft. x 50 ft. Run along the outside perimeter of this figure and count laps. Laps are converted to miles in Table A-1. Proceed as in step 4.

Results

1. On the basis of this test, what is your fitness category? _____

2. Are you pleased, satisfied, or dissatisfied with the results? _____

3. Do you believe that more experience in how to establish a pace would help improve your score? _____

4. Do you believe that this test accurately reflects your present level of circulorespiratory fitness? _____

LABORATORY 6

EVALUATION OF CIRCULORESPIRATORY FITNESS (HARVARD STEP TEST)

Name _____ Instructor _____

Class and section _____ Date _____

Purpose

The purpose of this laboratory session is to evaluate your circulorespiratory fitness by means of the Harvard Step Test. This test is based on the fact that the speed at which you recover from hard exercise is a reliable indicator of your level of circulorespiratory fitness.

Equipment Needed

1. One sturdy 20-in. bench; one sturdy 18-in. bench
    If gymnasium bleachers are to be used, 2-in. by 6-in. boards bolted into place on top of the seat increase the step height sufficiently to permit substitution for the 20-in. bench.
2. Metronome
3. Timer with a second hand that will run for 8.5 minutes consecutively

Procedure

The male subject steps up and down on the 20-in. bench 30 times per minute for 5 minutes. The female steps up and down on the 18-in. bench 30 times per minute for 4 minutes.

At the end of the test, the subject sits immediately. The pulse is counted and recorded during 30-second intervals after 1 minute, 2 minutes, and 3 minutes of recovery. Use the following score sheet to calculate your score for the test.

Recovery Period	Pulse Count
1 to 1.5 min.	_____
2 to 2.5 min.	_____
3 to 3.5 min.	_____
Sum of 3 pulse counts	_____

Long Form

$$\text{Index} = \frac{(\text{Duration of exercise in seconds}) \times 100}{2 \times (\text{Sum of pulse counts during recovery})}$$

$$= \frac{(\qquad) \times 100}{2 \times (\qquad)}$$

$$= \underline{\qquad\qquad}$$

$$\text{Index} = \underline{\qquad\qquad}$$

Short Form

$$\text{Index} = \frac{(\text{Duration of exercise in seconds}) \times 100}{5.5 \times (\text{Pulse count, 1 to 1.5 min.})}$$

$$= \frac{(\qquad) \times 100}{5.5 \times (\qquad)}$$

$$= \underline{\qquad\qquad}$$

$$\text{Index} = \underline{\qquad\qquad}$$

Classification

Below 55	Poor
55-64	Low average
65-79	Average
80-89	Good
90 and above	Excellent

Results

1. How do the results of this test compare with your performance on the 12-minute run? ＿＿＿＿＿＿

2. Which test do you perceive to be physically more demanding? ＿＿＿＿＿

3. Are you pleased or displeased with your score? ＿＿＿＿＿＿

CAROTID PULSE MONITORING AND TARGET HEART RATE DURING TRAINING

Name _____ Instructor _____

Class and section _____ Date _____

Purpose

The purposes of this laboratory session are to practice palpation of the carotid pulse, to determine how high you must elevate your heart rate to achieve a training stimulus, and to get a feel for a training pace that elicits your target heart rate.

Equipment Needed

Stopwatch or wristwatch with a second hand

Procedure

1. Use the first two fingers on your preferred hand to find your carotid artery. (See Figure 3-2, p. 28).
2. Press *lightly* until you can feel your carotid pulse.
3. Count your pulse for 10 seconds, then multiply by six to get your heart rate for 1 minute.
4. Try this several times during a 10-minute rest period while you are either seated or reclining.
5. Assume that the lowest value obtained is your resting heart rate, calculate your exercise target heart rate as follows.

			Example
a.	Predicted maximum heart rate*	= _____	200
b.	Resting heart rate	= − _____	− 70
c.	Maximum heart rate range	= _____	130
d.	Percentage of MHR range for training (60%, 70%, 80%)	= × _____	× 0.60
e.	Multiply step c times the desired value from step d	= _____	78
f.	Resting heart rate	= + _____	+ 70
g.	Target heart rate for training	= _____	148

*See Table 3-3, p. 29, for estimated maximum heart rate by age.

6. Now jog slowly for 3 minutes. Stop and *immediately* count your carotid pulse for 10 seconds.
7. If the intensity of the exercise was too light, the rate will be lower than the desired rate. If this is the case, jog a little faster for 3 more minutes and take your pulse rate again. Continue until you have found the pace at which you must work.

Results

Once you develop a feel for your own pace, you should be able to maintain the desired rate comfortably for 10 to 15 minutes. After a few training sessions, you will need to reexamine your resting heart rate to see if a new target rate is to be determined. In each training session, it is desirable to monitor your heart rate both during and immediately after the exercise to insure an adequate level of intensity for training.

INTERVAL TRAINING

Name _____ Instructor _____

Class and section _____ Date _____

Purpose

The purpose of this laboratory session is to demonstrate the use of interval (intermittent) training, as might be used indoors or outdoors in a relatively small area.

Equipment Needed

1. Timing device with a second hand, such as a wall clock, lab timer, stopwatch, or wristwatch
2. Marked area approximately 94 ft. x 50 ft. (the size of an official basketball court)

Procedure

Progress through an interval-style workout as outlined below. The work consists of a series of activities that are interspaced with recovery periods. The work will become progressively harder, will reach a peak, and then will taper off.

1. Begin with 3 to 5 minutes of stretching and flexibility exercises as described on pp. 54-71.
2. Walk two laps (2L) around the perimeter of the basketball court (or a 94-ft. x 50-ft. rectangle) at a vigorous pace.
3. Walk 1L at a vigorous pace while you make swimming movements with your arms.
4. Racing-walk ½L, then walk regularly the remainder of the lap.
5. Walk 1L vigorously with swimming arm-movements again.
6. Jog 1L very slowly.
7. Walk 1L to recover.
8. Jog 1L at a moderate pace (25 to 30 seconds per lap).
9. Walk 1L to recover.
10. Jog 1L at a moderate pace.
11. Walk 1L to recover.
12. Jog 2L at a moderate pace. Walk 1L to recover.
13. Jog 3L. Walk 1L to recover.

Note: *Check heart rate* during the *first 10 seconds* after jogging 3L and remember the value.

14. At center court, execute the following high-intensity exercises consecutively. *No rest intervals.* Exercises are to be executed *as fast as possible!*
    a. Running, in place, knees waist-high for 15 seconds
    b. 10 push-ups
    c. Repeat step a
    d. Supine flutter kicking for 15 seconds
    e. Repeat step a
    f. Prone flutter kicking for 15 seconds
    g. Repeat step a
    h. 10 sit-ups
    i. Repeat step a
    j. 10 squat jumps
    k. Repeat step a
    l. *Check heart rate immediately*
15. Walk 1L to recover.
16. Jog 3L at a moderate pace. Walk 1L to recover.
17. Jog 2L at a moderate pace. Walk 1L to recover.
18. Jog 1L. Walk 3L to recover.
19. Cool down for 5 to 10 minutes before a shower.

Results

This program produces varying degrees of stress depending on (1) how vigorously the steps are executed and (2) the physical condition of the participant. If your heart rate was below 130 or 140 beats per minute at the end of step 13, you should (1) increase the pace (e.g., to 20 seconds per lap) and (2) increase the number of consecutive laps (e.g., to 4L or 5L) before you proceed to the high-intensity exercises. After the high-intensity exercises (step 14) are completed, your heart rate should be at least as high as your target heart rate (75%) as calculated by Karvonen's method. (See p. 29.) In the early stages of training, most people prefer to interspace work with frequent rest periods. As your body adapts to the repeated stress over a period of days or weeks, you will need to increase the stimulus by (1) increasing the pace, (2) progressively increasing the number of consecutive laps, or (3) removing the recovery laps to make the program more continuous than intermittent.

CIRCUIT TRAINING FOR STRENGTH

Name _____ Instructor _____

Class and section_____ Date _____

Purpose

The purpose of this laboratory session is to demonstrate a modification of the classic circuit-training approach as applied to strength training.

Equipment Needed

1. A Universal Gym or some similar weight-training apparatus
2. A timer with a second hand (e.g., Gra-Lab timer) that will run for 30 minutes consecutively

Procedure

1. Determine the *maximum* amount of weight that can be handled through 5 repetitions (5 RM) of each of the following exercises.
   a. Leg curls
   b. Weighted chins
   c. Leg press
   d. Bench press
   e. Weighted sit-ups
   f. Military press
2. Begin with step 1a. Complete the 5 RM within 30 seconds; then rest for 60 seconds.
3. Proceed to step 1b. Repeat the 5 RM within 30 seconds and rest for 60 seconds.
4. Continue the pattern until all steps (a-f) have been completed three times (three sets). Note: In the second and third sets, initially you might not be able to complete 5 RM due to fatigue. As you increase in strength, you will find that you can do much beyond the initial 5 RM, particularly in the first set. To keep the work uniformly distributed over the three sets, you must adhere to the following regulations.
   a. *Do not exceed* eight repetitions in the first or second sets no matter how strong you feel.

b. If you execute eight repetitions in the first and second sets and you can exceed eight repetitions in the third set of a particular exercise, you must establish a new 5 RM for that lift. To find the new 5 RM, simply add weight until 5 repetitions are once again the maximum you can lift without a pause for rest.

c. Remember to stagger the lifts so that the same muscle groups are not used in successive exercises.

d. Remember to work on a 1:2 work-relief ratio (e.g., work 30 seconds if needed and rest for 60 seconds).

Results

This type of weight training is very strenuous and should be engaged in only triweekly on nonconsecutive days. As the resistance increases, you may need some slight assistance to overcome the inertia of a weight at rest.

BODY FRAME AND ACCEPTABLE BODY WEIGHT

Name _____ Instructor_____

Class and section _____ Date _____

Purpose

The purpose of this laboratory session is to estimate your body-frame size and acceptable body weight.

Equipment Needed

1. Measurement tape
2. Scales

Procedures

1. Estimate your body-frame size (small, medium, or large) with the technique described on p. 81.
2. Estimate your acceptable body weight with Table 6-2 (p. 80).
3. Use the OW index described on p. 81 to estimate whether you are overweight. Values of 100 or less are considered to indicate a good weight, and values greater than 110 are considered to indicate overweight.

Results

Acceptable body weight is best estimated through measurement of the percentage of body fat. Is your weight acceptable to you as compared with the standards given above?_____

Ankle girth measurement _____

Body frame _____

Weight _____

Height _____

OW index _____

ESTIMATION OF
BODY-FAT PERCENTAGE

Name _____ Instructor _____

Class and section _____ Date _____

Purpose

The purpose of this laboratory session is to estimate your percentage of body fat.

Equipment Needed

Skinfold calipers

Procedures

1. Have your skinfold thicknesses measured as described on pp. 81-84.
2. Use the appropriate formula on p. 184 to estimate your percentage of body fat.

Results

1. Use 15% for males and 20% for females as the upper normal limit of body fat. Are you satisfied with your percentage of

   body fat? _____

   Some individuals desire a lower percentage than the upper normal limit.
2. To estimate pounds of fat that exceed the desired amount of body fat (15% or 20%), use the following formula:

   Excess pounds = Body weight x (Percentage of body fat
   $\qquad$ − Desired percentage of body fat)

   Example: a male who weighs 210 lb. with 25% body fat desires to have 15% body fat.

   $$\text{Excess pounds} = 210 \times (0.25 - 0.15)$$
   $$= 210 \times 0.10$$
   $$= 21 \text{ lb.}$$

   This male has 21 lb. of fat in excess of his desired 15%.

SAMPLE CALCULATION OF PERCENTAGE OF BODY FAT

Step 1. Calculation of Body Density

For females,*

Body density = 1.0764
— (0.00081 x [Skinfold thickness at iliac crest])
— (0.00088 x [Skinfold thickness at triceps])

Skinfold Site	Sample Thickness[†]	Actual Thickness[†]
Iliac crest	13 mm	_____ mm
Triceps	10 mm	_____ mm

Body density = 1.0764 — (0.00081 x 13) — (0.00088 x 10)
= 1.057

For males, [††]

Body density = 1.1043
— (0.001327 x [Skinfold thickness at thigh])
— (0.001310 x [Skinfold thickness at scapula])

Skinfold Site	Sample Thickness[†]	Actual Thickness[†]
Scapula	11 mm	_____ mm
Thigh	11 mm	_____ mm

Body density = 1.1043 — (0.001327 x 11) — (0.001310 x 11)
= 1.0753

Step 2. Calculation of Percentage of Body Fats**

$$\text{Percentage of body fat} = \frac{4.570}{\text{Body density} - 4.142}$$

For the sample female,

$$\text{Percentage of body fat} = \frac{4.570}{1.057} - 4.142 = 0.182 = 18.2\%$$

For the sample male,

$$\text{Percentage of body fat} = \frac{4.570}{1.0753} - 4.142 = 0.108 = 10.8\%$$

*Sloan, A.W.; Burt, J.J.; and Blyth, C.S., Estimation of body fat in young women, *Journal of Applied Physiology* 17: 967-970, 1962.
[†]Average of two measurements.
[††]Sloan, A.W., Estimation of body fat in young men, *Journal of Applied Physiology* 23: 311-315, 1967.
**Brozek, J.; Grande, F.; Anderson, J.T.; and Keys, A.; Densitometric analysis of body composition; Revision of some quantitative assumptions, *Annals of the New York Academy of Science* 110: 113-140, 1963.

SEVEN-DAY RECORD OF CALORIC CONSUMPTION AND ENERGY EXPENDITURE

Name _____ Instructor _____

Class and section _____ Date _____

Purpose

The purpose of this laboratory session is to determine your caloric consumption and energy expenditure for a seven-day period.

Equipment Needed

None

Procedure

Maintain a record of your weight, food intake, exercise, and Calories expended for a seven-day period on pp. 186-192. Use Tables 6-8 (pp. 94-98) and 6-9 (pp. 99-100) for this purpose.

Results

1. Are your caloric intake and energy expenditure in balance? _____

2. Did you gain weight, lose weight, or maintain the same weight during the seven days? _____

3. Should you adjust your food intake and physical activity for good weight management? _____

SUMMARY OF TOTAL CALORIC INTAKE AND
EXPENDITURE THROUGH EXERCISE FOR SEVEN DAYS

Name _____ Body Weight _____ Date _____

Instructor_____ Course & Section _____

Date _____

Time   Food   Calories   Exercise & Calories Used

Date _____

Time	Food	Calories	Exercise & Calories Used

Date _____

Time	Food	Calories	Exercise & Calories Used

Date _____

Time	Food	Calories	Exercise & Calories Used

Date _____

Time	Food	Calories	Exercise & Calories Used

Date _____

Time	Food	Calories	Exercise & Calories Used

Date _____

Time	Food	Calories	Exercise & Calories Used

THE TENSE INDIVIDUAL

Name _____ Instructor _____

Class and section _____ Date _____

Purpose

The purpose of this laboratory session is to determine if you are a tense individual.

Equipment Needed

None

Procedures

1. Read each of the 25 questions listed below and answer them yes or no. Give the answer that describes you.
2. Have a friend answer the questions to reflect how he or she perceives you.

Results

Tense people seek to release their tension in physical actions that are in no way related to the problem created by the tension. If you answered yes to many of the questions listed below, you may need to reexamine your perception of the stressor, seek diversions to provide your worried mind with new problems that can be solved, participate in physical activity to provide a release for the tension, and participate in some form of relaxation technique. Answer each question yes or no.

Yes   No

_____   _____   1. Do you often experience headaches or backaches?

_____   _____   2. When sitting in a chair and talking to someone, do you continually move in the chair to seek a comfortable position?

_____   _____   3. When retiring for the night, are you unable to fall asleep immediately?

_____   _____   4. Do you often grind your teeth when you are confronted with an unpleasant experience?

Yes   No

_____   _____   5. Do you easily become angry or frustrated when you are faced with a problem for which there is no immediate solution?

_____   _____   6. Do you often complain of being tired?

_____   _____   7. Does your face often hold expressions of intense concentration?

_____   _____   8. Do you often drum your fingers aimlessly or forcibly to express irritation?

_____   _____   9. Does your posture appear stiff when you sit or walk?

_____   _____   10. Are you unable to concentrate on one problem at a time?

_____   _____   11. Are you unable to relax voluntarily?

_____   _____   12. Do you often experience nervousness and uneasy feelings?

_____   _____   13. Do you become upset when your plans are interrupted or must be changed?

_____   _____   14. Are you highly competitive in sports, in your test grades, and in your daily responsibilities?

_____   _____   15. Are you time-conscious?

_____   _____   16. Do you experience extreme dissatisfaction and anxiety when you fail to achieve success in your endeavors?

_____   _____   17. Are you an aggressive person?

_____   _____   18. Are you often too busy to allow time for physical activity?

_____   _____   19. Do you plan your day's activities and often budget your time?

_____   _____   20. Are you critical of yourself when you make a mistake?

_____   _____   21. Do you feel "uptight" at the end of the day?

_____   _____   22. Are you impatient when others are late for an appointment with you?

Yes   No

———— ———— 23. Do you often set high goals or levels of achievement for yourself?

———— ———— 24. Do you experience bad moods very often?

———— ———— 25. Are you unyielding when others disagree with your beliefs or convictions?

RELAXATION TECHNIQUES

Name _____ Instructor _____

Class and section _____ Date _____

Purpose

The purpose of this laboratory session is to practice the conscious release of muscular tension (relaxation). It is a skill that is not easily performed by many individuals.

Equipment Needed

1. Mats
2. Pillows or towels

Procedures

1. Practice the Benson relaxation technique described on p. 108.
2. Have a partner or group leader guide you through the Arnheim relaxation technique described on pp. 108-110.

Results

1. Did either of the relaxation techniques help you release muscular tension? _____

2. Do you need to develop the skill to consciously relax? _____

POSTURE EVALUATION

Name _____ Instructor _____

Class and section _____ Date _____

Purpose

The purposes of this laboratory session are to evaluate your posture when standing, walking, running for distance (jogging), and lifting a heavy object and to make you aware of postural mechanics that should be followed for each of these positions and movements.

Equipment Needed

None

Procedures

1. Wear a bathing suit if possible.
2. Work with a partner. Each evaluates the posture of each other.
3. Refer to the posture mechanics described on pp. 141-144 and use the evaluation forms in the Results section to estimate your partner's posture. Score each aspect of posture as follows: no deviation — 0; slight deviation — 1; moderate deviation — 2; extreme deviation — 3.

Results

Individuals who are not trained to do so may find it difficult to evaluate posture accurately, but this experience can provide insight into postural mechanics.

1. Are you pleased with your posture evaluation? _____

2. Should you practice better posture mechanics? _____

Standing (refer to p. 141)

1. Head and chin _____

2. Shoulders _____

3. Shoulder blades _____

4. Chest _____

  5. Trunk _____

  6. Abdomen _____

  7. Hips _____

  8. Arms _____

  9. Knees _____

 10. Feet _____

 11. Weight _____

Walking (refer to pp. 141-142)

  1. Upper body _____

  2. Trunk _____

  3. Motion _____

  4. Lead leg _____

  5. Base of support _____

  6. Supporting and pushing leg _____

  7. Lead heel _____

  8. Ankle joint of pushing leg _____

  9. Weight shift _____

 10. Leg muscles _____

Running for Distance (refer to p. 143)

  1. Head _____

  2. Back _____

  3. Buttocks _____

  4. Elbows _____

  5. Body _____

  6. Footstrike _____